Derrel R. Watkins, PhD, MSW, M.
Editor

Religion and Aging: An Anthology of the Poppele Papers

Religion and Aging: An Anthology of the Poppele Papers has been co-published simultaneously as *Journal of Religious Gerontology*, Volume 12, Number 2 2001.

Pre-publication
REVIEWS,
COMMENTARIES,
EVALUATIONS . . .

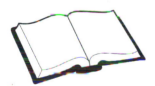

"**A** wonderful compilation of papers dealing with a subject that has been somewhat ignored by gerontologists! Professor Watkins' book is a must read for anyone currently ministering with older adults as well as those preparing for this growing area of ministry. Leaders of seminaries and theological schools will also find this book to be a valuable resource as they contemplate and implement curricular changes."

James L. Knapp, PhD
Associate Professor of Sociology
Southeastern Oklahoma State
University

More pre-publication
REVIEWS, COMMENTARIES, EVALUATIONS . . .

"**E**nlightening, comprehensive, insightful. An invaluable resource. Among the most valuable sections are those which deal with practical advice, ministry suggestions, and training needs. The more reflective sections cause one to ponder the crucial issues of aging through the lens of Scripture and thus offer peace and hope for an otherwise dismal period."

Martha S. Bergen, PhD
Associate Professor
of Christian Education
Hannibal-LaGrange College
Missouri

"**A** wide-ranging collection of essays . . . challenged my ministry with older adults and provided beneficial insights and practical suggestions. The chapter on using Psalms in nursing home ministry is fresh and perceptive."

Reverend Robert R. Phillips, BME, MM
Associate Pastor
First Baptist Church
Sedalia, Missouri

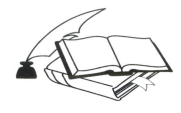

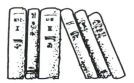

The Haworth Pastoral Press
An Imprint of The Haworth Press, Inc.

D19

Religion and Aging: An Anthology of the Poppele Papers

Religion and Aging: An Anthology of the Poppele Papers has been co-published simultaneously as *Journal of Religious Gerontology*, Volume 12, Number 2 2001.

Dementia Services
Development Centre
University of Stirling
STIRLING FK9 4LA

The *Journal of Religious Gerontology*^{TM} Monographic "Separates" (formerly *Journal of Religion & Aging*)*

Below is a list of "separates," which in serials librarianship means a special issue simultaneously published as a special journal issue or double-issue *and* as a "separate" hardbound monograph. (This is a format which we also call a "DocuSerial.")

"Separates" are published because specialized llibraries or professionals may wish to purchase a specific thematic issue by itself in a format which can be separately cataloged and shelved, as opposed to purchasing the journal on an on-going basis. Faculty members may also more easily consider a "separate" for classroom adoption.

"Separates" are carefully classified separately with the major book jobbers so that the journal tie-in can be noted on new book order slips to avoid duplicate purchasing.

You may wish to visit Haworth's website at . . .

http://www.HaworthPress.com

. . . to search our online catalog for complete tables of contents of these separates and related publications.

You may also call 1-800-HAWORTH (outside US/Canada: 607-722-5857), or Fax: 1-800-895-0582 (outside US/Canada: 607-771-0012), or e-mail at:

getinfo@haworthpressinc.com

Religion and Aging: An Anthology of the Poppele Papers, edited by Derrel R. Watkins, PhD, MSW, MRE (Vol. 12, No. 2, 2001) *"Within these pages, the new ministry leader is supplied with the core prerequisites for effective older adult ministry and the more experienced leader is provided with an opportunity to reconnect with timeless foundational principles. Insights into the interior of the aging experience, field-tested and proven techniques and ministry principles, theological rationale for adult care giving, Biblical perspectives on aging, and philosophic and spiritual insights into the aging process."* (Dennis R. Myers, LMSW-ACP, Director, Baccalaureate Studies in Social Work, Baylor University, Waco, Texas)

Aging in Chinese Society: A Holistic Approach to the Experience of Aging in Taiwan and Singapore, edited by Homer Jernigan and Margaret Jernigan (Vol. 8, No. 3, 1992) *"A vivid introduction to aging in these societies. . . Case studies illustrate the interaction of religion, personality, immigration, modernization, and aging."* (Clinical Gerontologist)

Spiritual Maturity in the Later Years, edited by James J. Seeber (Vol. 7, No. 1/2, 1991) *"An excellent introduction to the burgeoning field of gerontology and religion."* (Southwestern Journal of Theology)

Gerontology in Theological Education: Local Program Development, edited by Barbara Payne and Earl D. C. Brewer* (Vol. 6, No. 3/4, 1989) *"Directly relevant to gerontological education in other contexts and to applications in the educational programs and other work of church congregations and community agencies for the aging."* (The Newsletter of the Christian Sociological Society)

Gerontology in Theological Education, edited by Barbara Payne and Earl D. C. Brewer* (Vol. 6, No. 1/2, 1989) *"An excellent resource for seminaries and anyone interested in the role of the church in the lives of older persons. . . . must for all libraries."* (David Maldonado, DSW, Associate Professor of Church & Society, Southern Methodist University, Perkins School of Theology)

Religion, Aging and Health: A Global Perspective, compiled by the World Health Organization, edited by William M. Clements* (Vol. 4, No. 3/4, 1989) *"Fills a long-standing gap in gerontological literature. This book presents an overview of the interrelationship of religion, aging, and health from the perspective of the world's major faith traditions that is not available elsewhere . . . "* (Stephen Sapp, PhD, Associate Professor of Religious Studies, University of Miami, Coral Gables, Florida)

New Directions in Religion and Aging, edited by David B. Oliver* (Vol. 3, No. 1/2, 1987) *"This book is a telescope enabling us to see the future. The data of the present provides a solid foundation for seeing the* *future." (Dr. Nathan Kollar, Professor of Religious Studies and Founding Chair, Department of Gerontology, St. John Fisher College; Adjunct Professor of Ministerial Theology, St. Bernard's Institute)*

The Role of the Church in Aging, Volume 3: Programs and Services for Seniors, edited by Michael C. Hendrickson* (Vol. 2, No. 4, 1987) *"Experts explore an array of successful programs for the elderly that have been implemented throughout the United States in order to meet the social, emotional, religious, and health needs of the elderly."*

The Role of the Church in Aging, Volume 2: Implications for Practice and Service, edited by Michael C. Hendrickson* (Vol. 2, No. 3, 1986) *"Filled with important insight and state-of-the-art concepts that reflect the cutting edge of thinking among religion and aging professionals." (Rev. James W. Ellor, DMin, AM, CSW, ACSW, Associate Professor, Department Chair, Human Service Department, National College of Education, Lombard, Illinois)*

The Role of the Church in Aging, Volume 1: Implications for Policy and Action, edited by Michael C. Hendrickson* (Vol. 2, No. 1/2, 1986) *"Reviews the current status of the religious sector's involvement in the field of aging and identifies a series of strategic responses for future policy and action."*

Published by

The Haworth Pastoral Press, 10 Alice Street, Binghamton, NY 13904-1580

The Haworth Pastoral Press is an imprint of The Haworth Press, Inc., 10 Alice Street, Binghamton, NY 13904-1580 USA.

Religion and Aging: An Anthology of the Poppele Papers has been co-published simultaneously as *Journal of Religious Gerontology,* Volume 12, Number 2 2001.

© 2001 by The Haworth Press, Inc. All rights reserved. No part of this work may be reproduced or utilized in any form or by any means, electronic or mechanical, including photocopying, microfilm and recording, or by any information storage and retrieval system, without permission in writing from the publisher. Printed in the United States of America.

The development, preparation, and publication of this work has been undertaken with great care. However, the publisher, employees, editors, and agents of The Haworth Press and all imprints of The Haworth Press, Inc., including The Haworth Medical Press® and Pharmaceutical Products Press®, are not responsible for any errors contained herein or for consequences that may ensue from use of materials or information contained in this work. Opinions expressed by the author(s) are not necessarily those of The Haworth Press, Inc.

The Haworth Press, Inc., 10 Alice Street, Binghamton, NY 13904-1580 USA

Cover design by Thomas J. Mayshock Jr.

Library of Congress Cataloging-in-Publication Data

Religion and aging : an anthology of the Poppele papers / Derrel R. Watkins, editor.
    p. cm.
    "Co-published simultaneously as Journal of religious gerontology, volume 12, number 2 2001."
    Includes bibliographical references and index.
    ISBN 0-7890-1388-6 (alk. paper)–ISBN 0-7890-1389-4 (pbk : alk. paper)
    1. Church work with the aged. 2. Aged–Religious life. I. Watkins, Derrel R., 1935-

BV4435.R45 2001
261.8'3426–dc21   2001024984

Religion and Aging:
An Anthology
of the Poppele Papers

Derrel R. Watkins, PhD, MSW, MRE
Editor

Religion and Aging: An Anthology of the Poppele Papers has been co-published simultaneously as *Journal of Religious Gerontology*, Volume 12, Number 2 2001.

The Haworth Pastoral Press
An Imprint of
The Haworth Press, Inc.
New York • London • Oxford

Indexing, Abstracting & Website/Internet Coverage

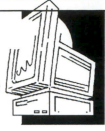

This section provides you with a list of major indexing & abstracting services. That is to say, each service began covering this periodical during the year noted in the right column. Most Websites which are listed below have indicated that they will either post, disseminate, compile, archive, cite or alert their own Website users with research-based content from this work. (This list is as current as the copyright date of this publication.)

Abstracting, Website/Indexing Coverage . . . . Year When Coverage Began

• *Abstracts in Social Gerontology: Current Literature on Aging* 1991

• *AgeInfo CD-Rom* 1994

• *AgeLine Database* 1994

• *Applied Social Sciences Index & Abstracts (ASSIA)*
    (Online: ASSI via Data-Star) (CD-Rom: ASSIA Plus)
    <http://www.bowker-saur.co.uk> 1994

• *ATLA Religion Database, published by the American*
    Theological Library Association <www.alta.com> 1991

• *BUBL Information Service, An Internet-based Information*
    Service for the UK higher education community
    <URL: http://bubl.ac.uk/> 1999

• *CNPIEC Reference Guide: Chinese National Directory*
    of Foreign Periodicals 1995

(continued)

(continued)

Special Bibliographic Notes related to special journal issues
(separates) and indexing/abstracting:

- indexing/abstracting services in this list will also cover material in any "separate" that is co-published simultaneously with Haworth's special thematic journal issue or DocuSerial. Indexing/abstracting usually covers material at the article/chapter level.

- monographic co-editions are intended for either non-subscribers or libraries which intend to purchase a second copy for their circulating collections.

- monographic co-editions are reported to all jobbers/wholesalers/approval plans. The source journal is listed as the "series" to assist the prevention of duplicate purchasing in the same manner utilized for books-in-series.

- to facilitate user/access services all indexing/abstracting services are encouraged to utilize the co-indexing entry note indicated at the bottom of the first page of each article/chapter/contribution.

- this is intended to assist a library user of any reference tool (whether print, electronic, online, or CD-ROM) to locate the monographic version if the library has purchased this version but not a subscription to the source journal.

- individual articles/chapters in any Haworth publication are also available through the Haworth Document Delivery Service (HDDS).

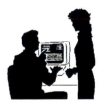

ABOUT THE EDITOR

Derrel R. Watkins, PhD, MSW, MRE, is Professor Emeritus of Social Work at Southwestern Baptist Theological Seminary, Oubri A. Poppele Professor of Gerontology (Retired) at the Saint Paul School of Theology, and currently serves as Adjunct Professor at the Institute for Gerontological Studies, Baylor University in Waco, Texas.

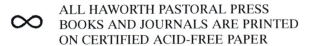

ALL HAWORTH PASTORAL PRESS
BOOKS AND JOURNALS ARE PRINTED
ON CERTIFIED ACID-FREE PAPER

Religion and Aging:
An Anthology
of the Poppele Papers

CONTENTS

Introduction

The *Quarterly Papers on Religion and Aging* were published by the Poppele Center for Health and Welfare Studies at the Saint Paul School of Theology in Kansas City, Missouri. The Poppele (pronounced pop-pel-e) Center was an endowed program funded by a generous grant from the estate of Miss Oubri A. Poppele, in 1979. The money was originally given to the United Methodist General Board of Global Missions for the purpose of establishing a center for training ministers for more effective health and welfare ministries, especially with older persons. Saint Paul School of Theology, located in the heartland of the United States, was chosen as the location for the center. David B. Oliver, a gerontologist and chair of the Department of Sociology at Trinity University in San Antonio, Texas, was employed as the first director. He was elected to the faculty as a tenured professor and provided oversight to the Poppele Center for Health and Welfare Studies. In 1984 the center printed the first issue of the *Quarterly Papers on Religion and Aging*. Rev. Nancy June Johnson served as the center director in the interim between 1990 and 1994. She edited the last issue that was published in 1994. The school closed the center and changed the focus of the professor/directorship to a full-time professorship. Derrel R. Watkins, Professor of Social Work at Southwestern Baptist Theological Seminary, was named to the Poppele Chair as Professor of Health and Welfare Ministries. Gerontology remained at the core of the professorship, but the *Quarterly Papers* were no longer published.

A wide range of scholars and students contributed articles for publication in the *Quarterly Papers*. Topics ranged from perspectives on aging from biblical and theological scholarship to practical pastoral

[Haworth co-indexing entry note]: "Introduction." Watkins, Derrel R. Co-published simultaneously in *Journal of Religious Gerontology* (The Haworth Pastoral Press, an imprint of The Haworth Press, Inc.) Vol. 12, No. 2, 2001, pp. 1-3; and: *Religion and Aging: An Anthology of the Poppele Papers* (ed: Derrel R. Watkins) The Haworth Pastoral Press, an imprint of The Haworth Press, Inc., 2001, pp. 1-3. Single or multiple copies of this article are available for a fee from The Haworth Document Delivery Service [1-800-342-9678, 9:00 a.m. - 5:00 p.m. (EST). E-mail address: getinfo@haworthpressinc.com].

© 2001 by The Haworth Press, Inc. All rights reserved.

1

emphasis on such ministry concerns as spirituality, nursing homes, alcoholism, preaching and other types of communication. In addition to articles written by David Oliver, scholars such as W. Paul Jones, Lindsey Pherigo, Nancy June Johnson, and Warren Carter from the Saint Paul School of Theology faculty were enlisted to contribute articles for publication. Other scholars such as Leo Missinne, Robert E. Buxbaum, James Ellor and Robert Coates, Barbara Payne, Justin P. Orr, and Susan H. McFadden also wrote scholarly articles that were published in the Quarterly Papers. Students such as Nanette Roberts, Elsie Tipton, LaDonna Carey, Pamela S. Hart, Sarah Hughes Haynes, and Amy Leeper contributed well-written articles as well.

This volume of the *Journal of Religious Gerontology* will not republish all of the articles. Some of the articles have been rewritten at the request of the original authors. Some are in process of being rewritten for submission at a later date. The articles that have been selected for this anthology are representative of those published in the *Quarterly Papers on Religion and Aging* during the ten years of its publication life. Many professors and students have expressed appreciation for the type of articles published in the Poppele Papers and have encouraged the *Journal of Religious Gerontology* to publish this edition.

Gerontology students at Saint Paul School of Theology assisted the editor in reading, selecting, and editing the articles included in this volume. Each of them made significant contributions to the process. Well over one hundred hours was spent on the project without a promise of a grade and with no financial remuneration. I wish to express my appreciation to each of them. Edar Rogler was especially helpful in coordinating the volunteer efforts of the group. She is both a practicing attorney and a student specializing in the study of gerontology. Colleen Williams is a chaplain at the Kingswood Manor Retirement Community in Kansas City, Missouri, specializing in gerontology on her Master of Divinity degree. Mari Berlin is a practicing nurse and a member of the Christian Church (Disciples) who is preparing for a ministry of Parish Nursing, especially with older persons. En He Han is a student from Korea who has already earned several advanced degrees, but he plans to complete the Master of Divinity degree with a concentration in gerontology and return to Korea and lead churches there in ministry with older congregants. Karen Lampe is a Presbyterian ministerial student specializing in gerontology in her theological studies.

The biographical information on each of the authors, for the most part, will reflect their positions at the time of their writing. Some have updated their biographical information and this will be included as well.

Derrel R. Watkins, PhD, MSW, MRE

A Holistic Approach to Ministry

David B. Oliver, PhD

Several years ago one of my students began working for a home-maker program. On her first visit she anxiously knocked on the door of her prospective client and was met by an elderly woman. The student said, "Ma'am, I'm from the City Homemaker Program and I'm here to help with your chores and the cleaning of your apartment." The woman appeared to be somewhat confused and irritated so the student went on to say, "Didn't the office call you?"

The woman, who later revealed her age as 85, looked carefully at the student and said, "Young lady! You're not here to help me! You're here to help Mother!" Sure enough "Mother" was 109 years old and all she really needed was someone to read *Newsweek* to her so she could keep in touch with the events of the world.

Due to tremendous advances in the treatment of chronic health conditions and the control of communicable and infectious diseases, more and more persons, like the woman in the story, are living to a ripe old age. During this century life expectancy in this country has skyrocketed to such an extent that persons reaching the age of 65 have a better than 50/50 chance of living well into their eighties.

The older segment of our population has experienced a period of

David B. Oliver occupied the Oubri A. Poppele Chair in Gerontology and Health and Welfare Studies at Saint Paul School of Theology. He holds a PhD in Sociology and Gerontology from the University of Missouri in Columbia. David is currently a member of the Health Sciences Faculty at the University of Missouri in Columbia, Missouri.

[Haworth co-indexing entry note]: "A Holistic Approach to Ministry." Oliver, David B. Co-published simultaneously in *Journal of Religious Gerontology* (The Haworth Pastoral Press, an imprint of The Haworth Press, Inc.) Vol. 12, No. 2, 2001, pp. 5-17; and: *Religion and Aging: An Anthology of the Poppele Papers* (ed: Derrel R. Watkins) The Haworth Pastoral Press, an imprint of The Haworth Press, Inc., 2001, pp. 5-17. Single or multiple copies of this article are available for a fee from The Haworth Document Delivery Service [1-800-342-9678, 9:00 a.m. - 5:00 p.m. (EST). E-mail address: getinfo@haworthpressinc.com].

© 2001 by The Haworth Press, Inc. All rights reserved.

phenomenal growth. This demographic explosion has had profound effects on various facets of our society including organized religion. While older persons have always been an integral part of our religious communities, only in recent times have they begun to represent the largest segment of the membership in churches, synagogues, and parishes. In fact, in some situations, particularly in rural areas, older persons represent anywhere from 50 to 100 percent of the total membership. Without question, organized religion in today's society is being confronted by significant challenges related to aging and the role of older persons within the church.

THE CHALLENGE OF AGING TO CHURCH AND SOCIETY

For centuries religious communities have struggled to bring value to those who were devalued. Yet we still have poverty, we still have racism, we still have fractured families, we still have hunger and we still have injustice. We have not found peace and we have not learned how to love our brothers and sisters in the household of God. Perhaps we should not be so presumptuous as to think that the outcome is any different with regard to the value accorded older persons.

Today Americans are preoccupied with the physical–the external characteristics of self. The pictures of what it means to be old so contaminate our thinking that we rarely risk going beyond the wrinkles to discover the soul.

Contemporary images of aging and oldness are dangerous, for they cause us to lower our expectations when we encounter older persons. If we see little value in the persons to whom we relate, the quality of our exchange with them has no chance to be anything more than disappointing. And, if we become so blind as not to recognize others as divine gifts, we deny us all the full drama of participation in the community of faith. Regardless of human condition we are loved from beginning to end. We are somebody. We count. We have value and worth all of our days.

In place of these wonderfully frail older persons, we can easily substitute other categories of rejected persons. For example, what about people with AIDS, the developmentally disabled, the homeless, the mentally ill, persons of color, orphans, and so on? We have a big job. We are up against *some* very big odds. And worse, the church we attend is not an inclusive one. Only socially acceptable people are welcome. Everyone is not invited to the banquet.

Acccptance comes at a very high price. If the church opens its doors, and its mission, to less-desirables in the community, it will more than likely lose some of its members. All we have to do is to observe the experience of old downtown churches once membered by the old aristocracy in our larger cities. Many of these churches are now referred to as "transition" churches. As less desirable people move in, the old guard moves out. Congregations are uncomfortable with people who are different. What they don't realize, of course, is that the problem is not with the socially unacceptable persons; the problem resides in them.

Why do we spend so little time with our elders? Why does the church continue to produce volume and volume and ream after ream of papers on children and youth when over half the membership is age sixty or older? Why do pastors talk about ministry to or for, rather than with, older persons? Why are older adults rarely thought of as persons in great need to evangelism–especially at a time when personal losses can occur in such rapid succession?

Why do family members collaborate with physicians and clergy before gathering information on the life worlds of their own loved ones? Why does the church seemingly disconnect the generations in its various programs and activities? Why are ministers so often out of touch with their own aging? Why is the subject of death constantly and inappropriately linked to aging? Why do we allow older persons to be dehumanized in our institutions?

All too often the church approaches older persons out of a sense of duty, with forced courtesy and undue sweetness, or with synthetic smiles and fabricated faces. If we could just realize that people in the latter third of life rarely ask for anything more than to be loved, recognized, included . . . to be a part of the community, the family, and the church.

The longer we live the more we find ourselves being abandoned by close friends and confidants. They die, they move away. In any event, we gradually are cut off from those who have, in the past, validated and reinforced who we are and with whom life has been a drama. Perhaps, it is at this time that the knowledge of God's continuous love–unconditional love–is more significant to our thinking, feeling, and acting than ever before.

We should be the first to reach out, latch-on, and make room for older persons so that they may bless our presence with their wisdom, experience, and stories. More than anything else, the church needs to open up to the sages of its older members. Only by listening to the lived moments of our elders will we ever be able to see the beauty of their being. God's presence in their souls will bless us again and again. Almost every time I am in ministry with an older person, I come away feeling as though it is I, rather than the other, who has been blessed by the experience.

We must expect and demand more of our opportunities to share fellowship with our elders. The church can become an extended family; utilize the experience, skills, gifts and graces of its elders; demand a stewardship on the part of its members which lasts a lifetime; be an advocate for its older members who have been dehumanized by secular systems; celebrate "redirection" rather than "retirement"; and be thankful for the servanthood, so frequently shown to us by the loving action of older members. But most importantly, the church can learn more about what it means to be part of the Kingdom by more fully incorporating aging persons in the midst of its ministry.

A HOLISTIC APPROACH

The challenges that confront today's church and society force us to develop a whole new conceptualization of oldness. What is aging? What does it mean to be older? How do we reconcile the vast difference between the social experience of growing old and the religious assurance that honor and respect accompany gray hair and wrinkles? How can wrinkles be valued?

Aging is much more than having birthdays. Older persons have spent years fine tuning, molding and carving out their unique personalities, characteristics and humanness. They are total human beings whose lives are created by blending of their physical and mental health, their social outlets and their spiritual insight. Thus, to theologize about what it means to be old requires that we examine the nature and process of aging along several dimensions.

PHYSICAL AGING

Physically, we all start aging in late adolescence. The process can speed up or slow down, and, thus, a great deal of variation may occur between and within persons. Most of us can expect to develop some health problems as we age. In fact, nearly 85 percent of older persons have one or more chronic health problems. However, we cannot make the mistake of beginning to assess our physical aging in terms of a medical chart. Rather, we must ask what a person *can* do; that is, how *functionally healthy* are they? Most older persons can function normally in spite of their health conditions.

An image of aging that over-emphasizes the physical dimension can get in the way of developing meaningful ministries with older persons. If we allow older members of our congregations to say, "I've paid my dues, let the younger people do it," we are not challenging them to stay active in their faith. Even among those who are less functional than others, we must challenge them to ask what they can do, rather than to dwell upon their limitations. Non-ambulatory stroke victims, who live in the wings of skilled nursing home facilities, have as much value and worth as those whose life circumstances are more fortunate.

In my view, practitioners and church members alike need to become less preoccupied with a "fix-it" mentality and shift to one of acceptance. After all, many suffering persons cannot be fixed. Only one out of two doctors will now follow their patient from the hospital to the nursing home (i.e., continue to be the patient's private physician). A major reason is their inability to "fix-it" (let alone diagnose it). As for acceptance, it is a subject that never gets taught in the professional school; therefore most doctors are uncomfortable with it. And so are ministers, and so are other practitioners . . . and so are you.

We must include all persons as divine gifts, whatever their physical state, as active participants in our religious communities. We are membered to them and must be open to what they can contribute to the community regardless–or perhaps because of–their human condition.

PSYCHOLOGICAL AGING

In order to understand the impact of psychological aging upon our lives we must ask ourselves the question, "What makes life a drama?" What makes life worth living? As we review the chapters in the story of our lives, what kinds of events stand out as most memorable? Generally, we celebrate our intimate, close, personal, relationships and events that we have shared with others. Rarely, do we recall our promotions or achievements or other material accomplishments.

Instead, we embrace those memories of the family reunion 20 years ago, or the funeral of a loved one, or the time on the mountainside when two people very much in love were sitting arm in arm watching the sunset and were one with God, one with nature, and one with each other.

Indeed, relationships make life a drama. Especially important are relationships with our close friends and confidants–those people who reinforce and validate who we are; in front of whom we stand naked; who know us so well we cannot wear a mask in their presence; and who love us in spite of who we are. Unfortunately, however, one of the realities which confronts us all is the fact that as we grow older our confidants die or they move away or lose their transportation and can no longer visit us, or they develop health problems which limit their participation in our lives.

What happens to us when our confidants are gone? Losing a confidant can be a tragic and painful experience. Most of us respond to such a loss by reaching out for someone else to love. We reach out to family, other friends, ministers, anyone who might love us in return. Usually this presents no problem if we are loveable and have a sense of humor and still get a kick out of life. But what if we are stroke victims whose lives and souls are locked inside very unlovable bodies?

Often when I visit a nursing home the administrator of director of nurses wants to introduce me to their favorite resident. Once I was visiting in a home where the "favorite" had just turned 100 years old and they were having a party and the news media were there. When they introduced me to her I leaned over and whispered in her ear, "Did they make over you like this when you were 99?"

"Hell, no," she whispered back, "I wish I had lied about my age." She was full of humor and delight to be around–she was lovable.

What about the unloveables? How can we relate to those who are paralyzed, incontinent, or whose appearance is dirty and unkempt? One of my students was called upon to visit a person in this condition. Later he confessed to me that he was thrilled and relieved to find the person asleep. And, as he was writing out a note to leave behind, he suddenly realized he was hurrying to complete it because the person might wake up.

The greatest fear of many older persons is the possibility of becoming unlovable and, as a result, being abandoned by family, friends, and even the church. Unfortunately, their fears are not unfounded. Many unloveables are abandoned and the only confidant they have left is God. And, sometimes, they may feel alienated from God's presence as well.

Assurance of God's love must be restored or reinforced. Practitioners, institutions, and congregations cannot continue to go their own way. They need to come together with a common purpose and a common goal. There needs to be a guiding force which not only unites all three in solidarity, but also one which motivates the kind of cooperative participation that builds community with and guarantees respect for the other.

If we are really concerned about an ethic of love, especially one informed by a theological stance which defines God as love, there would be a space on the planning chart specifying the name, address and phone number of the person who loves our resident the most. It would reveal the name of the confidant or close friend who can be counted on to show-up during difficult times. Can we identify which person *in* our facility is the closest to each resident? Is it the housekeeper? Is it an aide? Do we know? We cannot evaluate our effectiveness based on how well we meet the state's *requirements*; instead, we must develop and follow our own—we must look to our common ground. Bragging about being "the best" is often based on the wrong criteria! We need to establish an additional set of expectations. There are no prohibitions against it.

Churches need to support religious institutions of caring financially, with their resources, and personally, with their time. Institutions, by the same token, need to welcome and provide space and training for volunteers. We should be actively engaged in recruiting church members to the marvelous opportunities of ministry that await them. Indeed, institutions can help the church become more authentic.

One of the most important issues we face in the context of our religious communities is how to restore the connection between the unloveables and their Higher Powers. We need to help them feel wanted again—to be membered to the religious community. However, this cannot be accomplished through once-a-month activity programs. Certainly they are useful, but they simply do not provide an optimal setting for the development of close friendships and confidant relationships. Moreover, this kind of programming is not always accessible to everyone—and especially not to those persons who need it most.

The laity of religious communities must expand their contact–both in frequency and in quality–to the alienated, the homebound, the institutionalized and lonely.

A minister, rabbi or priest cannot do it all. We must remind ourselves that clergy and other religious professionals are not the only "minister." We are all called to ministry. If we do not claim a relationship with those to whom we are membered, we are doomed to frustration and failure. Our churches, synagogues and parishes can become extended families to those who are abandoned if we will only open up our lives to them. To be cut off from daily interaction with persons who love us is to experience a psychological death that is far worse than the physical one. God, working through us, can bring love back in the lives of the unloveables.

How can we help? How can we minister not only to those for whom we care, but also minister to those who leave to us the job of providing care for their loved ones. Again, *acceptance* is the key. We must teach family members, church members, professionals, and others who find our work amazingly difficult and depressing that while it is difficult at times, it is not depressing at all. We must teach them that, in the end, it is we that get blessed in this work. We receive it back ten-fold. The best-kept secret in working in caring institutions is the love we get in return for what we do.

SOCIAL AGING

In order to remain active in old age, good physical and mental health are prerequisites. This is one reason why many older persons are so preoccupied with them. To be physically fit and mentally alert in old age has become a status symbol even more so than a new car or a piece of property. Perhaps the significance of good health is reflected in the fact that physically active persons, regardless of age, are rarely perceived as "old." And, more importantly, these persons rarely perceive themselves as old.

An older person can, however, be physically and mentally fit, but trapped between the living room, bedroom, and kitchen twenty-four hours a day. Lack of transportation, a depreciated self-image, decreased vision and hearing, and a cluster of other problems may limit one's social world. Having nothing to do tomorrow, or the next day, or the next, can begin to diminish what good physical and mental health remains. We must do everything we can to extend warmth and affection from our religious communities to these individuals. Once contact is made–or once it has been restored–the ministry that follows must be *with* older persons. Doing things together, going places, sharing experiences–in essence, getting the person out of their daily living environment into the world of social involvement.

A sudden change in living environment can be particularly devastating for older individuals. To have to move from an eight to ten room house to an eight-by-ten room in a congregate living residence or nursing home is a major disruption of lifestyle. Future expectations, sense of security, predictability of events as well as visiting, eating and sleeping patterns, may all be affected. Waking to a quiet, peaceful morning broken only by the noise of chirping birds is quite different from waking to the noise, traffic and movement of staff and others in a nursing home. We often underestimate the trauma that a change of this sort brings to a person's life, even though we know that such a move is something we would abhor. As a defense mechanism to avoid feelings of guilt we deny this reality and, thus, leave little room for candid, honest, helpful discussion with persons who are involved in such a move. As a result, we automatically exclude ourselves from their social world.

To theologize about a person's existence requires an understanding of how that person lives, works and plays. Our assumptions may be totally misplaced if we cannot put ourselves in the midst of the other's world. It is critical that we enter the life-worlds of those with whom we hope to minister. We must get the story of who they are. This means leaving our own agenda behind. To listen carefully to others means to accord value and worth to their existence, to their being. We cannot possible get to know another person if we fail to hear the exciting chapters of their life.

It was Jesus who left the crowd to touch the leper, and who said, "When you do it unto the least of these, you do it unto me." We are speaking here of grace, of unconditional acceptance, of a Holy Love which both *transcends* and *transforms* human beings. It requires getting beyond ourselves to exist for the other. Only with a power greater than ourselves can we get beyond our own self-centeredness.

Acceptance is desperately needed within our institutional settings. Wanting everything to be all right and fixed is a problem. But ironically, it is in the institution that we can find role models of acceptance. I have seen more unconditional love being exchanged in a nursing home than in a church, and this from persons who are often the object of criticism, hate and hostility. Entry-level personnel: aides, house-keepers, and others who are the lowest paid and least trained persons on the staff, can teach us more about love and acceptance than other (more highly trained) persons in the organizational structure.

SPIRITUAL AGING

We are somebody, we are a gift, we are loved unconditionally, regardless of our place and condition. God's loving grace for each of us is a message that needs to be heard–and, more importantly, exper-ienced–by persons who feel alienated and abandoned. Some theolo-gians have called for a "theology of aging" when actually the old theology is just fine. We simply need to articulate it in direct concert with the experience and needs of older persons. Moreover, a kind touch transmitted through the holding of knowing and understanding hands can often be a sufficient expression that God still loves us. Theology of the best kind never needs to be spoken.

From the pulpit, however, the message and word of God does need to be made manifest. I am perplexed to find that many religious pro-fessionals seem to ignore older persons as potential recipients of evan-gelism. Yet there is never a more important time across the life span than the old age when God's unconditional love needs to be shared with persons who have been or who are experiencing a series of losses. Loss of health, loss of confidants, loss of income, loss of housing, loss of transportation, and so on, seem to come in accelerated pace. Many of these losses occurring over a short period of time can have a devastating effect on the individual. The need to feel membered is as important in old age as in earlier years.

After I preached a sermon entitled, "God as Confidant," an elderly widow approached me at the back of the church. As she thanked me for visiting and preaching on a topic so directly related to her, she glared at her minister standing next to me and said, "I have been a member of this church for nearly thirty years, and this is the first time a sermon has spoken directly to me!" With that, she gave me a kiss and went out the door. I haven't been invited back.

We must not avoid or deny the realities of aging that confront persons of all ages. We should question, however, whether or not we are overemphasizing youth at the expense of our older members. The stories in our sermons, the lessons in our Sunday School classes, and adult forums should all approach aging openly and honestly. The parables and many stories in the Bible lend themselves beautifully to the physical, psychological and social worlds of older persons.

All too often, however, the minister, rabbi or priest will bring in the psychologist, the social worker, the physician or some other expert to deal with aging concerns. This is unfortunate. Our religious professionals have as part of their training and experience many answers and more appropriate images of aging than any secular specialist can hope to bring. The Old Testament and New Testament clearly celebrate the value and worth of personhood in old age. Why can we not highlight these examples?

CONCLUSION

Aging along the four dimensions: physical, mental, social and spiritual, and the influence of each process on the other, must be conceptualized holistically. For example, let us say that, physically, you suffered a stroke. While a physical problem, it quickly becomes a psychological dilemma as you develop a negative self-image. Moreover, your physical appearance and psychological image combine to cause people to withdraw from you thus substantially reducing your social world. Consequently, you begin to feel abandoned–even by God. One lady in a nursing home once told me, "No, I haven't prayed in five years. I don't know who to pray to anymore."

It could be concluded from this holistic imaging of the aging process that "oldness" means being nonfunctional, having no confidants, experiencing a void in one's social world, and feeling spiritually dead. It should be pointed out that if this is the case, you can be "old" at any age. Indeed, any serious approach to religion and aging must focus on personhood and not age–age must be taken out of the equation. To minister effectively with older persons we must do our homework. We should ask: How functional is our friend? How many (if any) confidants provide love and support? What happens in his/her social world? Does he/she know and experience what it is like to have God taken up residence in his/her soul?

Our religious communities need to be more responsive to the value and worth of each individual, they need to respond more directly and effectively with the concerns of adult children who are perplexed about what to do with their aging parents, and every attempt needs to be made in terms of converting secular images of aging into more long-honored sacred ones.

TURNING TO A HIGHER POWER

I once thought that there was some magical formula for moving people to acceptance and all I had to do was find it. I was wrong. Only a power greater than ourselves can get us there. Only by turning over our uncomfortableness and the need to control things can we be liberated. When this first happens I think it sneaks up on us without warning. It's like one day we are miserable being cooped-up with these persons rejected by the larger society, and then the next day we look past their shortcomings directly into their souls and see the light. And it is brilliant. It is honest. It is loving. It is unselfish. And it is pure.

Perhaps God does reside in each of us, but it seems that only when we are at the most vulnerable point in our lives does it become abundantly clear. No wonder the poor will inherit the earth. And those who mourn will be comforted. The humble do receive what God has promised. And those who are merciful to others, receive mercy. The pure in heart do see God. And those who work for peace, are clearly God's children . . . part of the family . . . part of the household of God. Yes, the persecuted know God, and God knows them. And the common ground for all of these to whom God is gracious is vulnerability.

God takes up residence in the hearts, minds and souls of the people for whom we provide care. And it is there, that we too, can discover God . . . and do . . . everyday. What a joy!

We need to share the story. We cannot keep it a secret. Our task is to bring "outsiders" inside. One thing is certain. This spiritual transformation cannot happen if the church remains outside at a distance. We need to move it in, up close and personal.

My hope and confidence in the future comes from my association with persons who have experienced this transformation. You can *see* the change in their *eyes*, in their actions, in their demeanor . . . yes, in their comfortableness. They get hooked on their work. They get hooked on these wonderfully different people. They get less self-centered. They become liberated. They become new creations.

While God does the transforming, we must carry the message. The connection is the common ground. The responsibility is ours.

The holistic approach to understanding suggested here is just a start. I hope, however, that the church, synagogue and parish get their act together before I grow old. I want my community to begin to celebrate the diversity which exists among older persons, the wisdom of the years, the humor only older persons can bring, the value of experience and knowledge, the reality of sexuality in later years, the need for confidants, the opportunity for something to do, and to celebrate and acknowledge the value and worth of persons apart from their age. I want others to assess my functional health, the number of confidants I have, get into and understand my social worlds, and love me regardless of my situation. More than anything I always want something to do and someone to do it with.

Religion in Gerontological Research, Training and Practice

Barbara Payne Stancil, PhD

Religion has played a minor role in gerontological research to explain the aging process, in teaching about the social psychological behavior of normal aging, and in the aging network as a source of social psychological support of older people. It took the budget cuts of the 1980s to arouse the interest of the aging network in religious organizations as a major source (of resources) available to help continue their programs and services. Agencies faced with the necessity of developing cooperative programs with churches/synagogues found they had little research information or staff specialists in agency and church programming to guide them.

The treatment of religion by gerontologists is not consonant with the importance that older people place on religion in their lives. No other social institution outside the family in American society is more pervasive in the lives of older people than the church/synagogue. Furthermore, the involvement has been a long one. Social activity in religious context rates high in importance for most elderly and contributes to their life satisfaction and personal adjustment to old age.

Two levels of religion are involved in gerontological research, teaching/curriculum and practice: the individual and organizational.

Barbara Payne Stancil was Professor of Sociology and Director of the Gerontology Program at Georgia State University, Atlanta, GA. She is a United Methodist minister and is currently retired. She continues an active research and writing program from her home in Georgia.

[Haworth co-indexing entry note]: "Religion in Gerontological Research, Training and Practice." Stancil, Barbara Payne. Co-published simultaneously in *Journal of Religious Gerontology* (The Haworth Pastoral Press, an imprint of The Haworth Press, Inc.) Vol. 12, No. 2, 2001, pp. 19-28; and: *Religion and Aging: An Anthology of the Poppele Papers* (ed: Derrel R. Watkins) The Haworth Pastoral Press, an imprint of The Haworth Press, Inc., 2001, pp. 19-28. Single or multiple copies of this article are available for a fee from The Haworth Document Delivery Service [1-800-342-9678, 9:00 a.m. - 5:00 p.m. (EST). E-mail address: getinfo@haworthpressinc.com].

© 2001 by The Haworth Press, Inc. All rights reserved.

The individual level includes religiosity and the non-associational practices of religion in the everyday life of the older person. The organizational level includes the group memberships, social roles, supports, and activities available to older members.

This paper discusses the uses of religion at both these levels and some implications for the future.

RESEARCH

It has been over a decade since Heenan[1] referred to research on religion and aging as the "empirical lacunae." While there has been activity, research on religion and aging remains a fragmented and under-researched area. Indeed, there seems to be less gerontological research on religion now than in the 1960s. The latest work reporting social science research on aging, the *Handbook of Aging and the Social Sciences*,[2] does not include a chapter on religion as did the 1960 *Handbook on Social Gerontology.*[3]

Most social science research on religion has been on the individual level. It has focused on religiosity across the life course and the function of religiosity in personal adjustment to retirement and old age.[4] There have been few organizational studies other than those on membership and attendance. Maves and Cedarleaf made the first and only comprehensive attempt to study the relationship of churches to older people from 1946-1948.[5] Others studied the integration of older people within congregations[6] and the clergy's attitudes toward older people.[7,8] Currently, Tobin[9] is investigating cooperative efforts of churches and service agencies in meeting the need of the elderly.

RELIGIOUS VARIABLES

Social scientists may use religion as a dependent, independent or intervening variable. In gerontological research, religion has been used most frequently as a dependent variable, i.e., age affects changes in religious behavior and practice rather than religious practice affecting aging behavior. As a dependent variable most research showed that: (1) normal aging changes (retirement, widowhood, health) affect religious participation, practice and happiness;[10,11] (2) devotional practices and faith are affected by age.[12,13,14,15,16,17]

As an independent variable, religion has been used in research to explain the relationship between religiosity and adjustment to events of old age,[18] and to test the disengagement theory.[19] We found no studies that used religion as an intervening variable.

METHODOLOGICAL ISSUES

Most of the research has been cross-sectional, which limits the explanation of the relationship between aging and religion to the comparison of age groups at one point in time. Data from cross-sectional study cannot be used to explain changes in religious behavior due to the aging process. Gerontologists learned the lesson of this fallacy from the early cross-sectional studies on age and intelligence.

When Wingrove and Alston (1974) used a longitudinal design, they were able to show that the variations in church attendance were attributable to forces other than the aging process, such as cohort differences and period effects. Using longitudinal data from the Duke study, Blazer and Palmor[20] were able to show that age-related problems may influence participation in religious activities (church), even though religious attitudes and private practices remain stable.

Currently, most of the assumptions about religion and aging are based on cross-sectional studies made 10 to 30 years ago. At least replications of the studies would provide information about the religious practices of older cohorts in the 1980s.

The religious categories used in gerontological research obscure the pluralistic nature of American religion. Categories to report church membership and participation have been collapsed to the major faiths, Protestant, Catholic, Jewish, other. This classification fails to identify variations among Protestant religious bodies.[21]

Most of the survey research has reported religious practices and the meaning of religion among the elderly. None has reported how and in what ways religious groups and churches are a part of the everyday life experiences in the social, psychological and physical processes of aging.

Most of the research has surveyed individuals apart from the individual in institutional or organizational settings. An example of the latter is Zoot's[22] study of the effects of religious participation in a nursing home.

Other methodological issues are related to the need to evaluate the validity and reliability of research measures used in research in gerontology and the development of new measures. See Payne (1982) for a detailed discussion of these issues.[23]

FUTURE RELIGIOUS RESEARCH

There are social indications that religious research will increase in the future as churches respond to the rapid graying of their congregations and as need as aging networks increase for information to plan cooperative programs with churches. Current research information is insufficient for these purposes, or indeed, as a basis for future research.

Future religious research can be expected to include some of the following:

1. Cross-sectional national surveys on aging, using religion as a dependent variable to provide basic profile data. Since the U. S. Bureau of Census quit collecting religious data in 1957, social scientists have been forced to rely on NORC, Gallup and Harris National opinion survey data. Only recently[24] has the annual statistical report of the National Council of churches included an age breakdown of membership by denomination.
2. Longitudinal panels using religion as an independent variable to gain new knowledge about the relationship of religion to mental and physical health of older people, and the development of social support networks and links to the community.
3. Case studies of churches to describe the way the organizational structure, beliefs and policies, activities, rituals, etc., affect the everyday life of older members; and to understand how the decline in numbers of youth and the increase in numbers of elderly, particularly women, affect the organizational goals, programming and economic viability of churches.
4. Descriptive studies of differences in the types of organizational structures and beliefs of the many denominations and sects in American society, their regional distribution, human service policies and aging policies.
5. Demonstration and pilot studies to test modes of agency and church cooperative programs.

Most studies will continue to use religion as a dependent variable. But whether as a dependent or independent, researchers should be encouraged to use various intervening variables such as sex, race, marital status to explain the differential impact of religion on the different populations of older people.

RELIGION IN GERONTOLOGICAL TRAINING

Indications of the way religion is used in gerontological instruction are the treatment of religion in the major textbooks, curriculum offerings and course syllabi. Major texts[25,26,27] include short sections (3-5 pages) on religion. Atchley[28] and Ward[29] link religion with voluntary associations as the major organizations that tie most older people to the overall community. Hendricks and Hendricks[30] focus on the continuity and differences in the meaning of religion among older people. The textbook writers were limited by the paucity and the age of the research literature. Most of the research data cited were collected 10 to 30 years ago from cross-sectional surveys. The exceptions were Blazer and Palmor's[31] analysis of the Duke longitudinal data on religion and the Harris[32,33] reports for the National Council on Aging. Even with these limitations, it is strange that the data have not caused more stir about religion along the gerontological way. For example: (1) seventy percent of those over 65 assessed religion as very important in their lives and only 3 percent of the elderly said they had no religious preference;[34,35] (2) religious activity gradually declines with age but religious attitudes remain stable;[36] (3) less than 5-15 percent of older people participate in senior centers or groups, but 61 percent attend church regularly.[37,38]

Most courses in aging do not include religion as a major topic area. A review of the syllabi in the resource materials for teaching the sociology of aging issued by the American Sociological association revealed that only 3 of the 34 courses included sections on religion. These were all at the undergraduate level and none of the specialized courses was on religion.[39]

The reverse situation was found in seminaries and schools of theology, which had courses on religion, but not aging. From 1974 to 1976 the National Interfaith Coalition on Aging (NICA) surveyed 174 seminaries and schools of theology about the number and nature of courses directly or indirectly related to gerontology. They found that 100 of the 135 institutions responding offered at least one course with gerontology content, and 37 seminaries reported they had at least one course in which gerontology was a major thrust of the course. Most of the courses were of an applied nature, e.g., congregational pastoral ministry and counseling.[40]

To increase course offerings in seminaries, NICA secured funding from the Administration on Aging for a two-year project on Gerontology in Seminary Training (GIST). The project included: (1) three regional workshops for seminary faculty; (2) the development and implementation of a curriculum project by participating faculty; and (3) reporting on the project at a nation conference of innovative models for gerontological training of clergy and lay leaders. Faculty members from 4 seminaries participated.

The executive director of the Association of Theological Schools, Jessie Zeigler,[41] observed that as a consequence of the GIST program these 40 seminaries have reconsidered or considered for the first time their responsibilities for the preparation of ministers/clergy to reach the growing proportion of their congregations over age 65. The project was reported in a special issue of *Theological Education*. Although the full extent of the impact of the GIST project on seminary training is not known, some results were curriculum projects in about 40 schools, establishment of several Gerontology Centers, e.g., Saint Paul School of Theology, Boston University, and the Presbyterian School of Christian Education. Many seminaries have added gerontology to their curriculum.

In 1978 Georgia State University's Gerontology Center and the seminaries in the Atlanta metropolitan area offered a seminar on Religion and the Everyday Life of the Elderly. Students from the University and the seminaries met with pastors and lay persons as a part of the curriculum. From this successful experience, an ecumenical committee was established to plan further training in religion and aging and to develop comparative models of ministry with and for older people. In 1982 the second joint seminar on Religion and Aging was offered to develop innovative models of training and service between congregations, agencies, and older people. Another by-product of the first seminar was a joint graduate certificate program in gerontology between Georgia State University's Gerontology Center and the Candler School of Theology.

THE FUTURE OF RELIGION/AGING CURRICULUM

This area can be expected to grow in importance within career preparation in aging as the economic constraints continue, the proportion of older people increases and congregations respond to the graying of the churches and society. The proportion of church members over age 65 is already much higher than for the general population. Latest data from Yearbook of the Churches (1982) shows denominational variations from 11 to 43 percent of the church members are over the age of 65, with the greatest increase expected in the next 50 years.[42]

It may also be expected that special topic courses and modules within courses dealing with religion will become parts of career preparation in gerontology. This will provide professionals to develop programs with congregations.

PRACTICE

Churches/synagogues have been providing special services to the elderly longer than public agencies and the aging network. Churches have provided residential homes, "shut-in" care, specialized educational programs, and recreational activities that developed social support networks for older members. Furthermore, their efforts were not unrecognized by the Administration on Aging (AOA). The models of church programs developed in the 1950s were widely used by AOA as models of appropriate group activities for older people.[43] The Eighth Annual Southern Conference on Gerontology was on organized religion and the older person.[44]

The residential and nursing homes built and operated by religious bodies date from the 1930s, and many of them were built with Federal 202 housing loans. Butler and Lewis reported in 1977 that religious institutions supported 44 percent of all nonprofit homes and 14 percent of nursing homes, and they had their own self-imposed standards and certification process.[45]

Whatever the form, the rest of the 1980s and the 1990s will see the development of models of cooperative programming between agencies and churches at the local and national level and between religious bodies and agencies. Some of this is under way but is underreported and fragmentary.

CONCLUSION

This brief examination of the major uses of religion by gerontologists in research, training and practice has reflected the limited research on religion and aging at the individual and organizational level, some future uses of religion in each area have been suggested, and it has been predicted that gerontological interest in religion and aging will increase in this decade.

NOTES

1. E. R. *Heenan*, "Aging in Religious Life," *Review for Religious Research*, 1968, *27* (1968) 1120-1127.

2. R. Binstock, and E. Shanas, (Eds.), *Handbook of Aging and the Social Sciences* (New York: Van Nostrand, 1976).

3. C. Tibbitts, (Ed.), *Handbook of Social Gerontology* (Chicago: University of Chicago Press, 1960).

4. B. Payne, "Religiosity," in *Social Roles and Social Participation*, (Volume 2), (Eds.), D. J. Mangen and W. A. Peterson (Minneapolis: University of Minnesota Press, 1982) 343-353.

5. P. B. Maves and J. L. Cedarleaf, *Older People and the Church* (New York: Abingdon-Cokesbury Press, 1949).

6. D. Moberg, "The Integration of Older Members in the Church Congregation," in *Older People and Their Social World*, (Eds.), A. M. Rose and W. A. Peterson (Philadelphia: F. A. Davis Company, 1965) 113-124.

7. C. F. Longino and G. C. Kitson, "Parish Clergy and the Aged: Examining Stereotypes," *Journal of Gerontology, 31* (1976) 340-345.

8. D. O. Moberg, "Needs Felt by the Clergy for Ministries to the Aging," *Gerontologist, 12* (1975) 170-175.

9. S. Tobin, quoted in "Churches and Agencies Often at Odds in Aiding the Elderly, Study Finds," *Aging,* (1982) 46-47.

10. Caven et al., *Personal Adjustment in Old Age* (Chicago: Science Research Associates, 1949).

11. D. O. Moberg, "Religiosity in Old Age," in *Middle Age and Aging: A Reader in Social Psychology,* (Ed.) B. L Neugarten (Chicago: University of Chicago Press, 1968).

12. D. Blazer and E. Palmor, "Religion and Aging in a Longitudinal Panel," *Gerontologist, 16* (1976) 82-85.

13. Caven et al., *Personal Adjustment in Old Age* (Chicago: Science Research Associates, 1949).

14. Y. Fukuyama, "The Major Dimensions of Church Membership," *Review of Religious Research, 2* (1961).

15. H. L. Orbach, "Aging and Religion: A Study of Church Attendance in the Detroit Metropolitan Area," *Geriatrics, 16* (1961) 530-540.

16. C. T. O'Reilly, "Religious Practice and Personal Adjustment of Older People," *Sociology and Social Research, 42* (1957) 119-121.

17. R. Stark, "Age and Faith: A Changing Outlook as an Old Process," *Sociological Analysis, 29* (1968) 1-10.

18. D. O. Moberg, "Religious Activities and Personal Adjustment in Old Age," *Journal of Social Psychology, 43* (1956) 261-267.

19. C. Mindel and C. E. Vaughn, "A Multidimensional Approach to Religiosity and Disengagement," *Journal of Gerontology, 33* (1978) 103-108.

20. D. Blazer & E. Palmor, "Religion and Aging in a Longitudinal Panel," *Gerontologist, 16* (1976) 82-85.

21. L. Harris, The Myth and Reality of Aging in America (Washington, D.C.: National Council on Aging, 1975).

22. V. A. Zoot, "Religious Participation in the Nursing Home: Is It Therapeutic?", a paper presented at the Society for Life Cycle Psychology and Aging (Chicago: November 12, 1980).

23. B. Payne, "Religiosity," in *Social Roles and Social Participation*, (Volume 2), (Eds.), D. J. Mangen and W. A. Peterson (Minneapolis: University of Minnesota Press, 1982) 343-353.

24. C. H. Jacquet, *Yearbook of American and Canadian Churches* (Nashville: Abingdon Press, 1982).

25. R. C. Atchley, *Social Forces in Late Life,* 3rd edition (Beltmont, CA: Wadsworth Publishing company, 1980) 330-336.

26. J. Hendricks and C. D. Hendricks, *Aging in Mass Society: Myths and Realities*, 2nd edition (Cambridge, MA: Winthrop Press, 1981) 360-364.

27. R. Ward, The *Aging Experience* (New York: Lippencott, 1979) 255-258.

28. R. C. Atchley, *Social Forces in Late Life,* 3rd edition (Beltmont, CA: Wadsworth Publishing company, 1980) 330-336.

29. R. Ward, The *Aging Experience* (New York: Lippencott, 1979) 255-258.

30. J. Hendricks and C. D. Hendricks, *Aging in Mass Society*: *Myths and Realities*, 2nd edition (Cambridge, MA: Winthrop Press, 1981).

31. D. Blazer and E. Palmor, "Religion and Aging in a Longitudinal Panel," *Gerontologist, 16* (1976).

32. L. Harris, *The Myth and Reality of Aging in America* (Washington, D.C.: National Council on Aging, 1975).

33. L. Harris, *Aging in the Eighties: America in Transition* (Washington, D.C.: The National Council on the Aging, 1981).

34. L. Harris, *The Myth and Reality of Aging in America* (Washington, D.C.: National Council on Aging, 1975).

35. L. Harris, *Aging in the Eighties: America in Transition* (Washington, D.C.: The National Council on the Aging, 1981).

36. D. Blazer & E. Palmor, "Religion and Aging in a Longitudinal Panel," *Gerontologist, 16* (1976) 82-85.

37. L. Harris, *Aging in the Eighties*: *America in Transition* (Washington, D.C.: The National Council on the Aging, 1981).

38. E. Palmore, "United States of America," in *International Handbook on Aging*, (Ed.), E. Palmore (Westport, CT: Greenwood Press, 1980).

39. E. Palmore, ed., *Teaching Sociology of Aging* (Washington D. C.: ASA Teaching Resources Center, 1982).

40. T. C. Cook, *The Religious Sector Explores Its Mission in Aging* (Athens, GA: National Interfaith Coalition, 1976).

41. J. Zeigler, "Editorial Introduction to Gerontology in Seminary Training," *Theological Education, 16* (1980) 273-274.

42. C. H. Jacquet, *Yearbook of American and Canadian Churches* (Nashville: Abingdon Press, 1982).

43. A. B. Stough, *Brighter Vistas: The Story of Four Church Programs for Older Adults* (Washington, D. C.: U. S. Department of Health, Education and Welfare, Administration on Aging, 1965.

44. E. Scudder, *Organized Religion and the Older Person*, Institute of Gerontology Series, Volume 8 (Florida: University of Florida Press, 1958).

45. R. M. Butler and M. L. Lewis, *Aging and Mental Health: Positive Psychological Approaches*, 2nd edition (St. Louis: Mosby, 1977).

Ministry with the Elderly:
Training Needs of Clergy

James W. Ellor, PhD, DMin, DCSW
Robert B. Coates, PhD

One of the significant groups of people that every pastor needs to be able to engage through ministry is the elderly. While older persons constitute eleven percent of our society, they often make up a much larger portion of our congregations. Their needs vary as widely as their numbers. Some seniors are important participants in the power structure of the church; others seem to prefer to be left alone. While some of the older members of the church invest numerous volunteer hours, others seem to have insatiable needs. This diversity presents a significant challenge to those persons engaged in educating women and men for ministry. However, the critical question is, given the fact that students can't learn everything, which *should* be available to them to prepare them for their vocation?

In an effort to address the question of training needs to be considered when educating for ministry with the elderly, a survey of parish clergy was carried out. The purpose of this paper is to report on the

James W. Ellor teaches Counseling at National-Louis University. He is also Associate Director of the Center for Aging, Religion and Spirituality and Parish Associate of River Glenn Presbyterian Church. Robert B. Coates has taught Sociology at the University of Chicago, University of Utah and Valparaiso University. He has served a parish in Utah as a pastor in the United Church of Christ. He is currently retired and living in Minnesota.

[Haworth co-indexing entry note]: "Ministry with the Elderly: Training Needs of Clergy." Ellor, James W., and Robert B. Coates. Co-published simultaneously in *Journal of Religious Gerontology* (The Haworth Pastoral Press, an imprint of The Haworth Press, Inc.) Vol. 12, No. 2, 2001, pp. 29-36; and: *Religion and Aging: An Anthology of the Poppele Papers* (ed: Derrel R. Watkins) The Haworth Pastoral Press, an imprint of The Haworth Press, Inc., 2001, pp. 29-36. Single or multiple copies of this article are available for a fee from The Haworth Document Delivery Service [1-800-342-9678, 9:00 a.m. - 5:00 p.m. (EST). E-mail address: getinfo@haworthpressinc.com].

© 2001 by The Haworth Press, Inc. All rights reserved.

results of that survey and to suggest some of the possible ramifications of these data for seminary educators.

THE NEED FOR TRAINING

Clergy and laypersons have been concerned about the needs of the elderly for thousands of years. The significance of this group has increased since World War II with the advances of medicine and the increasing numbers of persons who are living longer. In 1940 a little more than six percent of the U. S. population was over the age of sixty-five.[1] Today, that number is nearly eleven percent.[2] These figures are even more dramatic for our churches. Comparison data is not available but our current research suggests that the average church or synagogue will have ten percent more elderly persons than is reflected in the local community.[3] Thus, if the community is consistent with the national average, thirteen percent of the population will be over the age of sixty-five; however, this means that the average church will have twenty-three percent of its members who are elderly. Among the predominantly United Church of Christ congregations reported in this study, these churches averaged thirty-one percent of persons over the age of sixty-five, with a range of 0-85 percent. While the reasons for these high percentages vary between congregations and denominations, some denominations including the Presbyterians and Episcopalians have reported that over fifty percent of their membership is over the age of fifty.[4] These figures suggest that the trend toward higher percentages of older person will continue in the future.

A second factor suggesting the importance emphasizing training for clergy and lay persons to work with the aged is suggested by evidence in the studies of Veroff et al. These writers suggest that the elderly, more than any other segment of our society turn to clergy first when they need emotional or other non-medical types of assistance.[5] Yet the role of the church and clergy in most communities is not that of a formal social service provider. Though many do provide some social services, the churches reflect what Berger and Neuhaus refer to as a "mediating structure," a natural or informal support.[6] As one pastor put it, "Our church is not in the business of providing social services, we are simply a family that is willing to help each other out." Whether the individual congregation is supplying formal social services, or informally acts to support its members, clergy and lay leaders in the church need to be aware of the fact that in many communities they have more consistent contact with the elderly than any other provider of services.

METHODOLOGY

In an effort to obtain a sample of parish clergy, two hundred names were taken from the graduation records of one Midwestern protestant seminary, closely affiliated with the United Church of Christ. Names of people were selected that either stated that they intended to go into the parish ministry, or people who identified specific churches that they would be working in upon graduation. These names were then checked against the current alumni/ae mailing list to obtain current mailing addresses for as many of the original group as possible. One hundred fifty-seven names and current addresses were obtained. A five-page instrument containing twenty-six questions was developed and mailed to all one hundred fifty-seven individuals. Seventy-four questionnaires, (47%) were returned for analysis.

CHARACTERISTICS OF RESPONDENTS

Analyses of the data suggest that the people who filled out this questionnaire are experienced in the life of the local church. Persons responding to this questionnaire graduated between the years of 1960 and 1983. Almost two-thirds (73%) graduated before 1976. Eighty-five percent are currently serving churches and ninety percent of the respondents have spent at least ten years in the local parish. The average pastor in this study is forty years old (ranging from 24 to 59). It is important to note that because the sample was taken from graduation records and because we cut off the sample with the class of 1959, none of the persons responding are themselves over the age of sixty-five. Twenty-three percent (17 of 74) are female and seventy-seven percent (57 of 74) are male. While the race of the persons selected for the sample was unknown to the person making the selection, ninety-six percent (71 of 74) of the persons who mailed the questionnaire back indicated that they were Caucasian with four percent (3 of 74) noting that they were Asian. The seminary from which the sample was drawn has a significant number of black graduates, yet there were not respondents that indicated that they were black.

When asked about additional training that prepared them for work with the elderly, twenty-eight percent (21 of 74) have attended workshops; fourteen percent (10 of 74) noted that they had attended continuing education courses. Eight percent of the persons filling out this questionnaire indicated that professional experience had contributed to their learning. (Multiple answers explain why the numbers do not add up to 74. Three persons did not answer this question.) Seven percent (5 of 74) of the respondents suggested that they had no training, and thirty-nine percent (29 of 74) did not answer this question. It is interesting to note that in Moberg's 1975 sample of 109 clergy, seventy-one percent of the persons responding stated that they had no specific preparation for ministry with older persons.[7]

A majority of the persons in this sample are from the United Church of Christ (50 of 71); fifteen percent (11 of 71) serve United Methodist churches; and eighteen percent (13 of 71) serve American Baptist, Roman Catholic, Church of God, Presbyterian, yoked churches and non-denominational congregations. (Three persons did not answer this question.) Sixty-nine percent (50 of 72) are the only ordained clergy person serving their church, while thirty-one percent (22-of 72) serve as a part of a multiple staff church. (Two persons did not answer this question.) The clergy in this sample average ten percent of their time with youth, thirteen percent with the elderly, twenty-six percent involved with worship, and twenty-five percent with administration. Twenty-six percent of their time is also spent with a variety of other tasks such as calling, counseling, studying, teaching, denominational work, and meetings.

The congregations served by the respondents are as diverse as the clergy themselves. Congregations average four hundred twenty-two persons, ranging from twenty-five to thirty-five hundred. These congregations average thirty-one percent persons over the age of sixty-five (ranging from 0 to 85%). The average income among congregants is $24,285 (ranging from $8,000.00 to $50,000.00). Eighteen percent (13 of 71) of the churches are in urban communities; thirty-five percent (25 of 71) are in suburban communities; thirty percent (21 of 71) are in small towns; seventeen percent (12 of 71) are in rural communities.

SKILLS NEEDED AND USED IN MINISTRY
WITH THE ELDERLY

Two types of content questions were asked of the respondents. The first group included questions about the skills necessary to work with the aged; the second group addressed questions about continuing education and ongoing support from the host seminary. Two primary questions were asked. The first asked how well the respondents felt they were prepared in various skill areas; the second asked how often they actually use the skills.

The findings suggest that empathy and small group leadership are the two skills for which the respondents felt best prepared. Long term counseling, social policy analysis, and family therapy lead the list for least prepared skills. It should be noted that several persons felt that empathy is not only an important skill essential to ministry, but that it was a gift of God. Examination of the use of skills suggests that preaching and empathy are the most frequently used skills, with leading small groups, program evaluation, and visiting the homebound also being frequently used. In contrast, psychological assessment, long term counseling, social policy analysis, analysis of individual social networks and family therapy are used less frequently. There is a strong association between the respondent's assessment of skills preparation and skills most frequently used.

A series of questions were also asked about the specific training available at the host school. The first question queried about the respondent's work with the elderly during seminary. Forty-eight percent (34 of 71) noted that they had successful experiences in the classroom. Courses included ministry, pastoral care, and house church. Thirty percent (21 of 71) also mentioned specific instructors that they found helpful. As one respondent put it, "Just knowing Dr. N. helped me to understand and work with the elderly." Fifty percent (36 of 71) noted either clinical pastoral education or field education as positive sources. (The 71 respondents indicate incomplete data.) These have traditionally been the sources of knowledge about ministry with the aged. Finally, twelve persons (17%) noted non-pastoral courses, continuing education activities, and personal experience. Eighteen persons (25%) said that they received no training to specifically work with the aged. This is in contrast with the study (done in 1974) by Moberg of one hundred and nine clergy where he found that seventy-nine percent of his sample had no specific training to work with the aged.[8] When asked about the most useful setting for the learning about ministry with the aged during seminary, forty-six (63%) indicated the classroom, and thirty-nine (54%) credited their field placement. A variety of pastoral care and ministry and nonministry courses were found to be useful.

When asked which skill areas should be emphasized in seminary, the following ranking was reported: listening (29%), assessment and referral (21%), knowledge of the changes in aging (20%), empathy (20%). Other key skill areas noted were family systems, calling, story telling, needs of the shut-in, patience, and death and dying.

When asked if there were specific skills needed that were not available in seminary, little consensus was obtained. While a lengthy list of pastoral care courses were listed, possibly the most interesting response was from the people who noted that even if the courses were available, they would not have had the time to take them.

Respondents were also asked how the training at the host school could be improved. Many people responded by listing specific courses on aging (22%), advocacy (13%), and ministry with specific age groups. Several people suggested formats, for example, sixteen percent of the respondents noted that ministry courses could be tied more closely to work in the local congregation. Others noted that they would have appreciated better advising on courses, particularly by persons from their denominations.

SIZE OF CONGREGATION AND SIZE OF STAFF

Working with a small sample seldom produces statistical trends of major significance. However, one trend that was derived from cross tabulation involved the number of persons on staff in the local church. When we compare churches with a single pastor with those with a multiple staff, the congregation size of churches with solo pastors is sixty-six percent fewer members. More to the point for this discussion, these small churches have a greater proportion of elderly members. And, their members have over five thousand dollars less per household upon which to live. When looking at skills identified as needed for working with the elderly, the solo pastor is somewhat more comfortable with empathy, counseling, assessment, small group analysis of social networks, analysis of social policy, visitation of homebound, and crisis intervention. While clergy who are part of a multiple staff church are at least somewhat more comfortable with referral, advocacy, program evaluation, community needs assessment, family therapy and conflict resolution.

These data reinforce the notion that the pastor who works for a multiple staff church has a different level of involvement with the aged. Multiple staff churches can afford to specialize in their ministry in areas such as work with the aged. However, the pastor who is the only ordained person on staff needs to be more the "jack of all trades." While solo work with more elderly persons, they generally cannot afford to hire even a semi-retired pastor to help with visitation.

If these data are consistent with the experience of other seminaries, the implications for education are that seventy-one percent of the graduates will be going to solo parishes, therefore needing a generalist education. The strength of the generalist is the ability to gain a few basic skills that can be used in a wide variety of situations. The generalist is unable to specialize in work with part of the congregation, because there is not anyone else to do the remaining tasks. Furthermore, a solo pastor likely has less per capita financial resources with which to do work. Some authors have suggested that clergy suffer from the same age biases as the rest of society resulting in less attention to the needs of the elderly. However, research has suggested that this is not true.[9] Possibly the reason that clergy are less involved in ministry with the aged has more to do with the realities of being the only pastor of a church than with ageism.

Skills clearly needed to work with the aged for the pastor who is the only ordained person in a congregation include the less technical, one-to-one skill of counseling, empathy, and visitation. The complexities of negotiating the social systems and advocating for large numbers of people's needs seem to be carried out more frequently by persons in multiple staff churches where more time can be spent attending community meetings and becoming involved with social agencies. We would caution that issues of time and size are important constraining variables. The church with only one pastor has less staff time to be able to devote to problems of a single group such as the elderly. Seminary education must take into consideration the needs of both pastoral settings.

CONCLUSION

Clergy have a long enduring relationship with the elderly. The aged are abundantly represented in many churches. Do these persons require a specialized ministry? How do clergy define the needed skills for work with the elderly? And, how do these clergy view their own seminary preparation for such work? These are some of the core questions dealt with in this report.

Listening to clergy concerns and ideas does not lead us to conclude that a highly sophisticated specialized ministry is needed in most churches. The minister is not usually expected to replace the social worker or the mental health worker. The needs of the elderly and the preponderance of elderly in our churches, however, do create a situation in which the elderly must be emphasized within a ministry to the total community.

Seminary education, as usual, walks a thin line of trying to prepare persons to develop ministries. While remaining committed to the traditional educational underpinnings of seminary education, the data presented above suggest that more material on needs of the elderly and applying generic pastoral skills with the elderly should be incorporated. These objectives can be achieved by emphasizing issues of the elderly in general pastoral courses and by adding selected courses focused on skill development for work with the elderly.

NOTES

1. M. W. Riley and A. Fonner, *Aging And Society* (New York: Russell Sage Foundations, 1968) 16.

2. C. S. Harris. *Fact Book on Aging* (Washington, D.C.: National Council on the Aging).

3. S. S. Tobin, J. W. Ellor, and S. M. Anderson-Ray, *Yearend Report* (An unpublished report to Retirement Research Foundation, 1982).

4. T. B. Robb, "Ministry with Grays", *Presbyterian Survey* (Vol. 21, 1981) 156-157.

5. J. Veroff, R. A. Kulka, and E. Donovan, *Mental Health in America*: *Patterns of Help-Seeking from 1957-1976* (New York: Basic Books, 1981) 156-157.

6. P. L. Berger and R. J. Neuhaus, *To Empower People*: *The Role of Mediating Structures in Public Policy* (Washington, D. C.: American Enterprise Institute for Public Policy Research) 26-33.

7. David O. Moberg, "Needs Felt by the Clergy for Ministries to the Aging," *The Gerontologist*, April 1975.

8. Ibid.

9. Charles F. Longino, and Gay C. Kitson, "Parish Clergy and the Aged: Examining Stereotypes," *The Journal of Gerontology*, 1976, Vol. 31. Number 3, 340-345.

Reflections on the Role
of the Church, Synagogue, or Parish
in Developing Effective Ministries
with Older Persons

David B. Oliver, PhD

From time to time, a number and variety of individuals, clergy and lay persons alike, have asked how the church/synagogue/parish might be more effective in developing ministries with older persons. I, too, have pondered this question. I have worked with congregations for a long time and have therefore experienced both successes and failures in working with the elderly. In this short piece I would like to share some of my reflections on do's and don'ts, and perhaps give some indication as to what is likely to work and what is likely to fail.

There is no particular significance to the order listed below. That is, I have not constructed an ordinal scale (suggesting that one item ranks higher than another), but rather I have simply listed some of the major things to consider if you plan to bring together older persons and ministry in any significant way.

1. Never consider a ministry *to*, or a ministry *for*, older persons. It is

---

David B. Oliver occupied the Oubri A. Poppele Chair in Gerontology and Health and Welfare Studies at Saint Paul School of Theology. He holds a PhD in Sociology and Gerontology from the University of Missouri in Columbia. David is currently a member of the Health Sciences Faculty at the University of Missouri in Columbia, Missouri.

[Haworth co-indexing entry note]: "Reflections on the Role of the Church, Synagogue, or Parish in Developing Effective Ministries with Older Persons." Oliver, David B. Co-published simultaneously in *Journal of Religious Gerontology* (The Haworth Pastoral Press, an imprint of The Haworth Press, Inc.) Vol. 12, No. 2, 2001, pp. 37-43; and: *Religion and Aging: An Anthology of the Poppele Papers* (ed: Derrel R. Watkins) The Haworth Pastoral Press, an imprint of The Haworth Press, Inc., 2001, pp. 37-43. Single or multiple copies of this article are available for a fee from The Haworth Document Delivery Service [1-800-342-9678, 9:00 a.m. - 5:00 p.m. (EST). E-mail address: getinfo@haworthpressinc.com].

© 2001 by The Haworth Press, Inc. All rights reserved.

much better to think in terms of a ministry *with* older persons, or better still, a ministry *from them* to the rest of us. This is perhaps best stated in the first issue of *Quarterly Papers* by W. Paul Jones (Vol. I, No. 1, Summer, 1984), "those who view life from the end can see uniquely into the heart of Being. Here we will find clues for ministry and an underlying 'new' spirituality." Indeed, it is my experience that the majority of older persons want to be included in the mainstream of church-synagogue/parish activities, not separated. And, they have much to bring to these encounters.

2. Never underestimate what your church synagogue/parish is already doing in the way of ministries with older persons. Every religious community in America has an aging program. Usually the persons who visit (and who are visited) are elderly themselves. These lay persons generally go about ministry very quietly but always consistently. They should be recognized, used as role models, and celebrated for the loving and caring they give to members of the congregation and to others in the community. Ministers and rabbis know who these persons are and are grateful for the service(s) they provide.

3. While some programs have been very successful in focusing exclusively on aging members themselves, if this is the only ministry involving the elderly, it would be a mistake. It serves to segregate rather than integrate older persons into the context of the church/synagogue/parish. Intergenerational programs should be encouraged along with the age-segregated activities. A good model of a natural and spontaneous intergenerational group is the choir. It usually has members of all ages, both sexes, meets at least twice per week (counting the Worship day), and most importantly, serves as a support group for those who participate. At any rate, most older persons do not want to be treated as some sort of special class. Instead, they want to experience an inclusive community–one to which they feel membered.

4. Ministers, rabbis, and lay leaders of religious classes need to ask themselves what scripture, experience, tradition, and culture have to say about older persons and the aging process. It is not always necessary to invite a gerontologist, social worker, nursing home administrator, etc., to bring the message about the elderly in our society. The church/synagogue/parish, indeed our faith, has much to offer on the subject. Thus, an intensive and intentional study of what our religious teachings and experiences say about aging is worth investigation–this does not require an outsider. The church/synagogue/parish should be

encouraged to do its own homework and bring to bear what resources the faith has to offer. The Old Testament is particularly rich in celebrating the value and worth of older persons. A starting point for an intentional study of faith and aging could be a Bible study program. The study could include an investigation into the stand your particular denomination and/or faith (at national and regional levels) has taken in response to religion and aging.

5. No successful aging program with which I am familiar ever got started by appointing a committee to organize it. Instead, the exciting programs which survive to this day were initiated by one or two persons dedicated to getting something started. Once begun, organization followed. It takes commitment and hard work. And, it usually helps if the person(s) doing the nitty-gritty are popular and respected by others in the religious community. The only limitation is one's imagination–anything is possible if you can only think of it and put it into action. Turning an idea over to a committee may quickly kill it.

6. While programs and activities that are leisure-oriented (that is, with a focus primarily on entertainment and relaxation) have their place, this should not be the major objective (or goal) of programming within the context of the church/synagogue/parish. Many older persons desire to be involved in mission, and if given an opportunity, particularly within the context of their religious community, they find more meaning and purpose in their lives. We retire people in the larger society, but we must not do it in the church/synagogue/parish. Stewardship and servanthood last a lifetime. Older persons who say "Pastor (or Rabbi), I've paid my dues, let the younger people do it," are missing opportunities to fulfill their purpose and role in the religious life. Even those who are less functionally healthy can participate if the religious leadership has the vision to see their continued value and worth. In short, "retirement" may be ubiquitous in the larger society, but it should be an unknown phenomenon in the context of the church/synagogue/parish.

7. There is no excuse for not having a telephone reassurance program. It is simple to put together and has many benefits. Making a list of who calls whom is just about all it takes. The organizer of the program will need to recruit and contact all the participants (in person if possible) and ask them what time of day would be best for them to receive and make a call. Then assignments are given. Content of conversation will vary according to the personalities involved, but it

can include church information, referral (services) information, and, most importantly, a friendly chat.

A church to which I was membered in San Antonio, Texas, was beginning to start a telephone reassurance program when one of our members was discovered in his home four days after he had died. He lived alone, and in his hand was clutched the telephone number of one of our parishioners. He died of a heart attack with the phone held tightly in his hand. Had our program been organized, he would have been discovered sooner by one of our callers. Short of death, a fall in the bathtub by a person living alone can be life threatening. Any caller who fails to receive an answer is always instructed to call a third party whose role it is to check the residence.

8. Every religious community should have a lay visitation program which guarantees that every nursing home resident, hospital patient, and homebound member gets a visit at least once (preferably twice) each week. This should be a one-on-one program, so the size of the group will depend on how many persons need visiting. The visitors need to meet at least once every two months (best once each month) to share stories, trade visitees, and build group solidarity. To avoid burn-out, volunteers know that they become a visitor for a designated period of time (usually one year), and then are assured that they will have a break from it. The lay visitation group should have a name and be well-known by all members of the church/synagogue/parish. One should receive high statue by being a member of it.

I have seen too many persons who have been abandoned by their religious family upon entering a nursing home to think that the church/synagogue/parish should do anything less. In fact, one measure of how well a religious community is doing is to ask how many of its less active members fail to get a regular visit from others members. One is too many.

9. Regular committees and planning groups need to be intentionally made up of persons of all ages. Every opportunity should be taken to insure an inclusive community. And, any program or activity involving older persons should most definitely have older persons as leaders and as planners. The Shepherd's Center concept, originating in Kansas City, has shown beyond any doubt the value of utilizing the skills of older persons to plan and implement exciting multidimensional programs.

10. Gatherings in small groups, even if this requires dividing larger

ones, is best. Older persons need to be able to share their stories and know that there are others who will listen. Many older persons feel as if no one listens to them anymore. This can quickly lead to a low sense of self-esteem, value, and worth. The church/synagogue/parish should provide opportunities for sharing, and therefore caring. Large impersonal groups simply reinforce superficiality. A close personal relationship (particularly with an individual of the opposite sex) has been shown to contribute, more than anything else, to higher morale and life satisfaction among older persons. The community of faith needs to facilitate opportunities for more meaningful encounters of this kind.

11. One-time events are interesting, but have no long-lasting effect. Don't limit our potential. Any serious attempt to respond to ageism in America, and issues surrounding adult children and aging parents, should be addressed throughout the congregation. As Ross Snyder suggests, our approach to aging needs to be "transgenerational." All members and categories of members in the church/synagogue/parish need to examine the processes of aging from each of their unique perspectives. Hopefully, significant and meaningful responses will follow.

12. The minister, priest or rabbi should not be the main force which organizes and sustains a ministry involving older persons. It should be a lay ministry. Professional leadership should encourage and facilitate innovative ministries, but because of tenure issues, the laity is in a better position to insure greater continuity and history. A program which rests on the charisma of a priest, rabbi or minister is in jeopardy when the clergyperson is transferred or moves on to another setting.

13. If persons are concerned about insurance and property before personal and human needs their hearts are in the wrong place.

14. Involve both men and women. Although women will outnumber men, be careful not to let a group become too female-dominated. If you do, you will lose the men. In old age, sexism gets turned upside down, and it is the old man who becomes the recipient of discrimination. It is particularly difficult to get widowers to return to religious activities following the death of a spouse. Programming needs to intentionally consider ways to attract and engage them. In one setting it is successfully done with pool tables. Again, you are only limited by your imagination.

15. Don't make your programs complicated. Keep them simple and meaningful. People should be more important than agendas. And,

don't schedule activities at night (early evening in the summertime would be okay).

16. Develop a variety of programs. Each older person is a unique individual with unique hobbies, interests, etc. If you put all of your eggs into one basket, you will miss many persons who would otherwise get involved.

My wife and I have two sons, ages 19 and 17. Already, they are two very different personalities. Moreover, they will go to different universities, select different occupations, marry (if they get married) into different families, join different interest groups, and have different friends and associates. By the time one is 80 and the other is 78, you may not be able to tell that they are brothers. Church/synagogue/parish programmers need to be alert to these basic differences. Older persons are not alike; each has his or her own set of needs and experiences. Do your homework.

17. Most programs should have a beginning and an end. Don't make them appear to last forever. You need to give people a chance to bail out gracefully.

18. Terminology can be very important. James McKay, a friend and distinguished psychologist, organized and advertised a special class about older persons and called it, "Mental Health and Aging." No one showed. He changed the title to "The Psychology of Happiness." This time there was a full house. Terms like "senior citizen" can turn people off as well. Ed Sinclair, a graduate of Saint Paul School of Theology, was once confronted with a long list of possibilities ("senior citizen," "older person," "the elderly," "the aged," "older adult," etc.) and quietly replied, "I prefer 'Sir' or 'Ma'am.'" Perhaps the best strategy is to recommend labels that make little reference to oldness and age in the first place. This would not be a form of denial; young persons have the same problem when others use stereotypical labels which serve to isolate and demean them.

19. Don't simply copy programs which have been successful in the secular world. Religious programming should be different *because* it originates within the context of the Christian or Jewish faith. To quote W. Paul Jones again, "To forge a religious ministry to the 'aging,' one must begin with the fundamental question–what difference does one's RELIGION make to the issue of gerontology? If religion simply adds a more kindly approach to doing what one would do anyhow from a

secular understanding of aging, religion is best eliminated from the field."[1]

20. Start small. Don't try to develop a multidimensional program involving a host of subprograms, objectives, and goals. Develop them one at a time. If you cannot pull off a one-dimensional (highly focused) program, then you surely will not be successful with a more ambitious one.

If you are considering doing more with all the talent, wisdom, experience, and knowledge in your congregation, you may find these twenty suggestions useful. The list is by no means exhaustive. I suggest that you use it as a starting point. You may wish to use them as a stimulus to group discussion and proceed from there.

NOTE

1. *Quarterly Papers*. Vol. I, No. 1, Summer, 1984.

Adult Children and Elderly Parents: The Worlds of the New Testament

Warren Carter, PhD

One of the points of continuity between the Hebrew Bible and the New Testament concerns care and respect for the elderly. The New Testament evidences this concern in diverse ways. Our focus will center on care for aging parents by adult children.

In requiring that adult children care for their aging parents, there is little doubt that the early Christian communities were influenced by the fifth commandment. New Testament writers quote the commandment "Honor your father and mother" in its Septuagint wording (Eph 6:2-3; cf. Exod 20:12; Deut 5:16). They cite it along with other commandments from the Decalogue (Mk 10:19) and refer to it as a commandment of Moses (Mk 7:10).

In our time, the fifth commandment is frequently understood as exhorting younger children to obey their parents. A number of scholars have recognized, however, that in both ancient Israel and in the early Christian Communities, this commandment addressed adult Children in multi-generational households.[1] It required from them a life-long obedience to and care for aging parents.

This understanding of the fifth commandment as requiring adult "children" to care for their aged parents is evident in several first-cen-

Warren Carter is Associate Professor of New Testament at Saint Paul School of Theology in Kansas City, Missouri. He received his PhD in New Testament at Princeton Theological Seminary.

[Haworth co-indexing entry note]: "Adult Children and Elderly Parents: The Worlds of the New Testament." Carter, Warren. Co-published simultaneously in *Journal of Religious Gerontology* (The Haworth Pastoral Press, an imprint of The Haworth Press, Inc.) Vol. 12, No. 2, 2001, pp. 45-59; and: *Religion and Aging: An Anthology of the Poppele Papers* (ed: Derrel R. Watkins) The Haworth Pastoral Press, an imprint of The Haworth Press, Inc., 2001, pp. 45-59. Single or multiple copies of this article are available for a fee from The Haworth Document Delivery Service [1-800-342-9678, 9:00 a.m. - 5:00 p.m. (EST). E-mail address: getinfo@haworthpressinc.com].

© 2001 by The Haworth Press, Inc. All rights reserved.

45

tury Hellenistic Jewish writers such as Philo and Josephus. We will briefly consider Philo's discussion, which discloses how some Jewish people understood the commandment when the Christian movement was beginning. Then we will note some similarities between Philo's discussion and other considerations of child-parent relationships in the Greco-Roman world.

PHILO AND THE FIFTH COMMANDMENT

Philo, who lived from about 30 BCE to 40 CE,[2] was a contemporary of Jesus and Paul.[3] He lived in Alexandria and participated actively in its large Jewish diaspora community. In a treatise, *The Special Laws*, he discusses the Ten Commandments and other Jewish regulations and practices. Scholars have seen a double purpose in this work. One purpose is to show the Gentile world how admirable and universal are Jewish laws and customs as set out, for instance, in the Pentateuch. Another purpose is to instruct Jewish readers about those things, which constitute Jewish identity and way of life in the midst of a dominant Gentile society.[4]

Philo begins his discussion of the fifth commandment by noting the God-like role of parents.

> The duty of honoring parents..stands on the borderline between the human and the divine. For parents are midway between the natures of God and man, and partake of both the human obviously because they have been born and will perish, the divine because they have brought others to birth and have raised not being into being. Parents, in my opinion, are to their children what God is to the world, since just as He achieved existence for the nonexistent, so they in imitation of His power, as far as they are capable, immortalize the race. (*Spec. Laws* II.225)

Philo finds further reason for honoring parents in the hierarchical nature of the parent-child relationship. Parents have superior virtue because of their age.

> Now parents are assigned a place in the higher of these two orders, for they are seniors and instructors and benefactors and rulers and masters: sons and daughters are placed on the lower

order for they are juniors and learners and recipients of benefits and subjects and servants. (*Spec. Laws* II.226-7)

Philo discusses the roles of parents as instructors and benefactors. They have provided life, education and daily necessities for their children at considerable cost. By the order of nature parents have authority over their children. This authority means "upbraiding and admonishing" children with words, beatings, putting them "in bonds," and, if necessary and by the agreement of both parents, putting them to death (II. 232,242-48). Nowhere in this discussion does Philo recognize that the nature of the relationship between parents and their offspring, a relationship of instruction and obedience, of beneficence and honor, of senior and junior, of older and younger, changes as children become adult children.

In addition to obedience, honor for parents is evidenced in other ways. "Courtesy shown to persons who share the seniority of the parents" is one way. Philo sees parents as "prototypes" of other elderly people. It is proper to be in awe of those who share one's parents' age.

The one who pays respect to an aged man or woman who is not of his kin may be regarded as having remembrance of his father and mother. (*Spec. Laws* II.237)

Philo cites some scriptural support for and examples of respect for the aged. Referring to Leviticus 19: 32, he sees the scripture requiring the young to give up seats to the aged and to yield to them as they pass.

A further part of Leviticus 19 attracts his attention. He notices that in verse 3 the lawgiver (Moses) instructs the young to "fear" their parents but omits to instruct them to "love" them. Philo finds this "admirable" because it is appropriate to Moses' purposes. Love or affection is learned by instinct. But those in need of instruction, "those who are in the habit of neglecting their duty," are those "wanting in sense, and want of sense is only cured by fear." Philo gives an example of children (the scenario points to adult children) who take what their parents give them as the basis for a life of extravagance and the indulgence of their lusts. Even with adult children, parents must actively and severely "cure the wastage of their children." The children must learn to be "in awe of those who begot them, fearing them both as rulers and masters" if they are to "shrink from wrongdoing" (Spec. Laws 11. 239-41).[5]

THE NON-JEWISH HELLENISTIC WORLD

What is striking about Philo's exposition of the fifth commandment is that much of the rationale for honoring parents is very similar to other discussions of parent-children relationships and of household organization found in non-Jewish (and non-Christian) writers. But these discussions are not based on the fifth commandment. Rather, they draw on a tradition of debate about household management that stretches back to Aristotle. By the end of the first century of the common era, the time of writing for many New Testament documents, the nature of household structures (including parent-children relationships) had been extensively debated for at least four hundred years since Aristotle (d. 322 BCE).[6]

In his work *Politics*, Aristotle discusses the State. He considers such matters as types of constitutions and government, what constitutes a citizen, the virtuous life, the goals, methods and subjects necessary to educate the ideal citizen. He begins his treatise, though, by arguing that households are the basic unit of any city or kingdom.

> And now that it is clear what are the component parts of the state, we have first of all to discuss household management; for every state is composed of households. (1.2.1)

Aristotle's initial tasks are to define the "household," and to identify how a household functions. He outlines four aspects of household management.

> The investigation of everything should begin with its smallest parts, and the primary and smallest parts of the household are master and slave, husband and wife, father and children; we ought therefore to examine the proper constitution and character of each of these three relationships. . . . There is also (another) department . . . the true position of which we shall have to consider: I mean what is called the art of getting wealth. (1.2.1)

For Aristotle, the household consists of three sets of relationships centered on the male. These relationships are marked by a hierarchical power arrangement. The husband, father, and master rules over his wife, children, and slaves.

> And since, as we saw, the science of household management has three divisions, one the relation of master to slave, of which we have spoken before, one the paternal relation, and third the conjugal for it is a part of the household science to rule over wife and children (over both as over freemen, yet not with the same mode of government, but over the wife to exercise republican government and over the children monarchical); for the male is by nature better fitted to command than the female (except in some cases where their union has been formed contrary to nature) and the older and fully developed person than the younger and more immature. (1.5.1)

By this definition, the household is androcentric (centered on the head male), patriarchal (marked by his rule over *his* wife, children, and slaves), and ageist (the older rule the younger). A fourth aspect, the male's task of accumulating wealth for the household (1.2.2), completes the four elements of the household.

The rule of father over children has several dimensions. The father rules "by virtue both of affection and of seniority" (1.5.2). He also rules because as an adult male he is naturally superior in virtue to children who are immature and imperfect in virtue (1.5.9).

While Aristotle requires the obedience of children to their parents, he does not discuss it in detail in the *Politics*.[7] However, while discussing friendship in the *Nicomachean Ethics*,[8] he identifies some important aspects of this relationship. Several times he compares the friendship of children and parents with that between people and the gods. Both are relationships to something "good and superior,"

> The affection of children for their parents, like that of men for the gods, is the affection for what is good, and superior to oneself; for their parents have bestowed on them the greatest benefits in the cause of their existence and rearing, and later of their education. (*NE* 8. 12.5)

Philo employs this thought some three hundred years later. Children remain obligated to their parents throughout their lives, unable ever to repay their father for all the benefits. But that does not offer adult children an excuse to withhold care from their parents. Aristotle knows that only a "bad son" will avoid aiding his father, or not eagerly undertake that task (*NE* 8.14.4). Adult children are to care for their parents. For example,

> It would be felt that our parents have the first claim on us for maintenance since we owe it to them as a debt, and to support the authors of our being stands before self-preservation in moral nobility. Honour also is due to parents, as it is to the gods. (*NE* 9.2.8)

As with Philo, such care for and honoring of one's parents throughout their lives is part of a general respect for the elderly in Aristotle's world.

> We should pay to all our seniors the honor due to their age, by rising when they enter, offering them a seat, and so on. (*NE* 9.2.9)

A TRADITION OF DISCUSSION

Aristotle's work predates the New Testament writings by some four hundred years. Nevertheless, Aristotle's ideas continued to circulate so that they were influential in the late first-century when the New Testament documents were written, and remained influential even beyond the time of the New Testament. Repeatedly this understanding of the household structure as forming the basis of the state, as consisting of the four elements (marriage, children, slaves, gaining wealth), and as being hierarchical, androcentric and ageist, is elaborated.[9] Such extensive discussion indicates that this understanding of the household structure was pervasive throughout the life and social experience of the ancient world.[10] It can be noted at this stage that this household structure is evident, for example, in Ephesians 5: 22-6: 9, in Colossians 3: 18-4: 1, and in a significantly revised form, in Matthew 19-20.

HIEROCLES: "ON DUTIES"

From early in the second century of the Common Era comes an interesting example of this tradition in the work *On Duties*, written by the Stoic, Hierocles.[11] Writing some four hundred years after Aristotle, a hundred years after Philo, and just a few years after most of the New Testament documents, Hierocles discusses human duties to the gods, to one's country, parents, friends, relatives and spouse. His consideration of duties to parents is informative in two respects. In contrast to the *general* emphasis in the household tradition on children respecting their parents, Hierocles' discussion offers particular insight with its description of specific duties and requirements. Further, like Philo, he offers a rationale for the actions and duties, thereby making explicit the cultural scripts informing the relationship.

Central to Hierocles' instructions about duties to parents is the recognition of a child's never-ending obligation to care for them. These duties are carried out in the context of daily life within the household. He thus addresses adult children in relationship to their aging parents.

> But we must begin with the assumption that the only measure of our gratitude to them is perpetual and unyielding eagerness to repay their beneficence, since, even if we were to do a great deal for them, that would still be far too inadequate.

He calls parents "the images of the gods, and . . . domestic gods, benefactors, kinsmen, creditors, lords and the firmest of friends." The meaning of parents as "images of the gods" is seen in Hierocles' description of how parents function:

> They guard our homes and live with us and are, furthermore, our greatest benefactors, supplying us with the most important things. . . . They are our nearest kinsmen and the causes of our relationship with other people. . . . They are, indeed, most justly our lords. For whose possession would we rather be than those through whom we exist? Moreover they are constant and unbidden friends and comrades . . .

The close identification between parents and the gods, a theme present in both Aristotle and Philo, supplies Hierocles with a memorable metaphor to express what is required of adult children.

> We should acknowledge that we live in our father's house as if we were attendants and priests of sorts in a temple, appointed and consecrated by nature itself, and entrusted with our parents' care.

For Hierocles, children must care for the bodies and the souls of their aging parents. With respect to care for their parents' bodies:

> We should liberally provide food for them which is adapted to the weakness that comes with old age, and in addition, bed, sleep, unguents, a bath, clothing, in short, all bodily necessities, so that they may never want for any of these things.

In supplying one's parents' physical needs, Hierocles sees adult children imitating the care that parents showed to them as newly born children. He extends the analogy to suggest that just as parents have to guess from "inarticulate and sobbing sounds" what the child needs, so adult children should try to discover their aging parents' needs "whether they mention them or not." There is a direct link for Hierocles between the quality of childrearing by parents and the care given subsequently to these now elderly parents by their children. In raising their children, parents "have become our teachers, instructing us in what they deserve to receive from us."

With regard to care for the "soul" of their aging parents, cheerfulness or joy comprises the greatest gift adult children can give.

> We should first afford them cheerfulness . . . by associating with them night and day, and as we walk, are anointed, and live with them. . . . Parents who are about to depart from life are particularly gratified by and hold dear the close attention their children pay them.

Cheerfulness also results from the manner in which adult children interact with their parents. Parents are not to be rebuked, but exhorted,

> Not as though they had erred in ignorance, but as though through inattention they had committed an oversight, which they certainly would not have committed, had they been more attentive.

Concern by adult children for their parents' physical needs also contributes to the parents' joy. For Hierocles, children function as servants to their parents,

> By performing even seemingly servile duties such as washing their feet, making their beds and standing ready to wait on them.

The children's love for those whom the parents consider highly provides a further source of joy:

> Children should therefore love their parents' relatives and consider them worthy of care, as they also should their parents' friends and in fact all whom they hold dear.

In a subsequent part of *On Duties*, Hierocles makes a similar point in discussing relationships with kinsfolk.

> The person who loves his kindred must treat his parents and brothers well and, on the same analogy, also his older relatives of both sexes, such as grandfathers or grandmothers, and uncles and aunts.

Hierocles is adamant that children are born and raised for the purpose of bringing their parents, especially their aging parents, joy and material provisions. Children are the insurance policy for their parents' (and grandparents') old age. In a subsequent section on "marriage," he names this purpose as the primary justification for the procreation of children.

> In the first place, then, we should consider that in children we not only beget for ourselves helpers, persons who will take care of us in our old age, and who will share with us in every fortune and circumstance; we beget them not only on our own behalf, but in many ways also for our parents. For the procreation of children pleases them since, if we should suffer some calamity before they die, we would leave them someone to take care of them in their old age.

By producing children, a couple also fulfills the wishes and hopes of their own parents. The continuation of one's family line ensures further honor and joy for parents.

> For from the first they attended to our birth, intending to have a very large issue and to leave behind a succession of children's children, and they planned our marriage, procreation and rearing. Hence, by marrying and begetting children we shall, as it were, answer part of their prayers, but, if we hold contrary opinions, we

shall thwart their deliberate choice. Moreover, it appears that everyone who voluntarily and without some prohibiting circumstance declines to marry and beget children accuses his parents of madness, as not having examined marriage with right reasoning.[12]

CONCLUSION

We have explored, briefly, understandings of the relationship between adult children and aging parents in several writings of the world from which the New Testament writings originate. While the fifth commandment was clearly important in guiding New Testament communities, we have observed an extensive Hellenistic tradition of discussion about household management including care for parents which, as I will now demonstrate, also seems to have impacted New Testament writers, but in different ways.

THE WORLD OF THE NEW TESTAMENT AND CONTEMPORARY QUESTIONS ABOUT AGING AND THE ELDERLY

Attention to this particular aspect of the culture from which the New Testament documents originated raises some interesting questions about the impact of this world on the early Christian communities. With respect to this household tradition and its requirement of utmost loyalty to one's parents, especially one's father, it is clear that Christian communities were impacted in different ways. Consider the following New Testament uses of this household structure we have been examining briefly. I will cite several NT writings, which probably originated at the same time, in the 80s of the first century.

From Matthew's gospel emerges a critique of this pervasive hierarchical household structure.[13] In chapters 19-20, successive sections are devoted to marriage relationships (19: 3-12), children (19: 13-15), acquiring and using wealth (19: 16-30), a parable about a householder (20: 1-16), being a slave (20: 17-29). In each case Jesus opposes the patriarchal household by urging "one flesh" marriage relationships, blessing children and identifying all disciples as children, redistribut-

·ing wealth in a more egalitarian manner, and calling all disciples to live as servants. While Matthew does not overthrow the command-ment to care for one's parents (15: 3-9; 19: 19), he envisions a new community in which the duty of adult children to their parents is not supreme.[14] Jesus' call to follow him, for example, literally overrides responsibilities to one's family and parents. James and John leave their father and the family fishing business (see Matt 4: 20-22).[15] Jesus redefines the household and family in terms not of birth but of doing the will of God (12: 46-50). The gospel writer refuses to absolutize the four-part, hierarchical, household structure and its pattern of parent-children relationship evident in the dominant culture. The new com-munity or family is constituted not by the pervasive androcentric and patriarchal pattern (cf. 23: 9), not by one's gender or age, but by one's commitment to God encountered in Jesus. This commitment creates in Matthew's gospel a more egalitarian, inclusive family structure, the community of disciples (12: 46-50) in which all disciples are children (19: 14) and servants (20: 25-26), and in which no human takes the role of an autocratic father (23: 9). This is a bold and daring call to a new community whose basis, focus and structure are in tension with a fundamental aspect of the first-century social fabric.

Yet a very different way of interacting with societal structures and values is evident in some other Christian writings about household structures. In Colossians and Ephesians, the writers adopt and advo-cate the Aristotelian household tradition as God's will for the Christian community (Col 3: 18-4:1; Eph 5: 21-6: 9). Husbands are to rule over wives, masters rule over slaves, and children are to obey their parents according to the fifth commandment (Eph 6: 1-3; Col 3: 20). In this model the Christian community imitates, not critiques, the dominant culture.[16]

Likewise in 1 Timothy 5, the Aristotelian tradition is carefully upheld as God's will. Young people are not to "speak harshly to an older man but speak to him as to a father" (1 Tim 5: 1-2). The (adult) children and grandchildren of a widow "should first learn the religious duty to their own family and make some repayment to their parents; for this is pleasing in God's sight. . . . And whoever does not provide for relatives, and especially for family members, has denied the faith and is worse than an unbeliever" (1 Tim 5: 4,8).

Clearly these texts do not speak with one voice about the relation-ship of children and parents. These writings present different patterns of interaction with the values and structures of their society. While they both uphold the fifth commandment, they do so in quite different ways because the writings do not place the same value on the pervasive household structure of the dominant culture.

And nor do they seem to speak equally. While we may admire the instruction to care for widows, we cringe at the instructions about slavery. And we know in the abuse that has resulted from teaching husbands to "rule over wives." Moreover, in the instructions to care for widows, there is some indication that a patriarchal agenda is being worked out, that, in the view of the author, some older women need to be controlled and domesticated so that they will not exercise leadership in the church, the preserve of men (1 Tim 5: 14-16; 4: 1-7; 3: 1-2,4-5, 11-12).[17]

The awareness of the diverse impact of societal values and structures on these NT writings urges contemporary readers, particularly those concerned with the very real and practical questions of aging and the elderly, to be cautious and informed in the task of interpretation.[18] In reading the New Testament we eavesdrop on the first-century dialogue about what it means to be Christian in a world that lives by very different commitments. The NT communities continually wrestle with the issue of being first-century people shaped by their society yet also formed by the good new of God's redeeming action in Jesus Christ.

As twenty-first century Christian readers, we are invited to join that dialogue and to share the same struggle to be faithful to our polyvalent traditions in ways that are appropriate to our particular cultural contexts. Realizing that it is a dialogue, that we enter a process of wrestling with diverse traditions, means that we will not demand of the biblical material what it cannot give us, namely, an instant, monolithic, neatly-packaged answer. Further, we enter that dialogue with the biblical material as people shaped by our world, experiences, questions, agendas, and participation in a community of faith, just as the NT texts are shaped by their world. At stake in the dialogue is to discern what God requires us to be as the people of God with respect to this particular issue in our time and circumstances.

The diversity of the NT material complicates the interpretive process in another way. This very diversity, of course, requires and enables us to choose one option rather than another. But it is also important to be sensitive to the tension that the canon creates in placing disparate material together in one collection of sacred writings. For instance, for today's "sandwich generation," the NT mandate to care for one's aging parents can come as an unwelcome and inconveniencing word in the midst of busy schedules, career goals, the quest for personal fulfillment, and the celebration of individual freedom. This mandate, if we pause long enough to reflect on it, raises complex questions about competing priorities and accepted societal commitments. But, on the other had, Matthew refuses to make the mandate to care for parents the supreme or only principle by which decisions should be made. That position is given to the claim of God's reign over our existence. When taken together, these quite different emphases in the canonical material create boundaries and tensions, which allow for various Christian responses to this situation.

These issues form a part of the complex nature of the task of exploring the presentation of aging and the elderly in the New Testament.

NOTES

1. See G. Blidstein, *Honor Thy Father and Mother: Filial Responsibility in Jewish Law and Ethics* (New York: Ktav, 1975); W. Harrelson, *The Ten Commandments and Human Rights* (Overtures to Biblical Theology; Philadelphia: Fortress, 1980) 92-105; J.G. Harris, *Biblical Perspectives on Aging: God and the Elderly* (Overtures to Biblical Theology; Philadelphia: Fortress, 1987) 61-64: S. Sapp, *Full of Years: Aging and the Elderly in the Bible and Today* (Nashville: Abingdon, 1987) 81-88. For some wider implications, C.J.S. Wright, "The Israelite Household and the Decalogue: The Social Background and Significance of Some Commandments," *Tyndale Bulletin* 30 (1979) 101-124, esp. 112-120.

2. In this article I shall use BCE (Before the Common Era) instead of BC, and CE (Common Era) instead of AD.

3. Citations of Philo are taken from F.H. Colson (trs.), *Philo* vol. 7, (Loeb Classical Library; Cambridge/London: Harvard University/Heinemann, 1958) 447-459. A helpful discussion of *Philo* is found in R. Williamson, *Jews in the Hellenistic World: Philo* (Cambridge: Cambridge University, 1989).

4. See, for example, Colson, *Philo*, General Introduction, xiv-xv.

5. It should be noted that another of Philo's works, *The Decalogue* 165-67, has a brief section on the fifth commandment which is essentially a summary of the points made in the much longer discussion in *Special Laws*. Another first-century Hellenistic Jewish writer, Josephus, has some brief comments on the fifth commandment in his work *Against Apion* written about the year 100 CE. While space precludes a consideration of Josephus, readers can observe how similar are his emphases.

> Honor to parents the Law ranks second only to honor God, and if a son does not respond to the benefits received from them—for the slightest failure in his

duty towards them–it hands him over to be stoned. It requires respect to be paid by the young to all their elders because God is the most ancient of all. (*Against Apion* II.206, from H. Thackeray, *Josephus* vol. 1 [Loeb Classical Library; Cambridge: Harvard University Press, 1961] 377).

6. Aristotle, *Politics* (Loeb Classical Library; Tr.H. Rackham; Cambridge: Harvard University Press, 1950).

7. For discussion of the immense power of the father over children in the ancient world (*patria potestas*), see J. Plescia, "*Patria Potestas* and the Roman Revolution," in S. Bertman (ed.), *Conflict of Generations in Ancient Greece and Rome* (Amsterdam: B.R. Gruner, 1976) 143-69; and W.K. Lacey, "*Patria Potestas*" in B. Rawson (ed.), *The Family in Ancient Rome* (Ithaca: Cornell University, 1986) 121-14. The first-century Stoic philosopher Musonius Rufus addresses the question of limitations to this power in "Must One Obey One's Parents Under All Circumstances?" in C. Lutz, *Musonius Rufus*: "*The Roman Socrates*" (New Haven: Yale University, 1947) 100-107.

8. Aristotle, *The Nicomachean Ethics* (Loeb Classical Library; Tr. H. Rackham; Cambridge: Harvard University Press, 1962).

9. The discussion of the Aristotelian model can be traced from Aristotle through the *Oeconomica*, the *Magna Moralia* (2nd Cent. BCE), Phildemus' *Peri Oikonomias* (1st Cent. BCE), Arius Didymus' Epitome (1st Cent. BCE), Hierocles" *On Duties* (early 2nd Cent. CE). It is also evident in the Neopythagorean works of Callicratidas, Occelus, Perictyone, Phintys (1st Cent. BCE-CE), in the *Antiquities* of Dionysius of Halicarnassus (1st Cent. BCE), in the Stoics Seneca, Epictetus, Dio Chrysostom (1st Cent. CE), and in the Hellenistic Jewish writers Philo, Pseudo-Phocylides and Josephus (1st Cent. BCE-CE). SeeD. Balch, "Household Codes," in *Greco-Roman Literature and the New Testament*, ed. D.Aune (Atlanta: Scholars, 1988) 25-50; D. Balch *Let Wives Be Submissive*: *The Domestic Code of 1 Peter*. (SBLMS 26; Chicago: Scholars, 1983).

10. In making this claim, I am aware that our evidence derives primarily from written, philosophical works authored by a educated elite. Evidence from across the social strata and from various geographical regions would no doubt introduce some modifications. However, the concession that the world and the household were never as neatly or as ideally structured as some of the writers would like, does not mean that this philosophical tradition is not reflective to some degree of actual structures.

11. See the translation in A. Malherbe, *Moral Exhortation, A Greco-Roman Sourcebook* (Philadelphia: Westminster, 1986) 85-104, esp. 91-93,97,103-4.

12. Hierocles offers a further justification for having children, to secure the future of one's state or country. See Malherbe, *Moral Exhortation*, 104.

13. For more detailed discussion, see W. Carter, *Households and Discipleship*: A *Study of Matthew 19-20* (JSNTSup 103; Sheffield: Sheffield Academic Press, 1994).

14. See S. C. Barton, *Discipleship and Family Ties in Mark and Matthew* (SNTSMS 80; Cambridge: Cambridge University Press, 1994) 1-56, 125-219.

15. W. Carter, "Matthew 4: 18-22 and Matthean Discipleship: An Audience-Oriented Perspective," *Catholic Biblical Quarterly* 59 (1997) 58-75.

16. See the more extensive discussion in Harris, *Biblical Perspectives*, 76-87.

17. See J. Dewey, "1 Timothy," in C. Newsome and S. Ringe (eds.), *The Women's Bible Commentary* (London/Louisville: SPCK/Westminster John Knox Press, 1992) 353-58.

18. W. Carter, "Matthew 4: 18-22 and Matthean Discipleship: An Audience-Oriented Perspective," *Catholic Biblical Quarterly* 59 (1997) 58-75.

The Psalms as a Resource
for Nursing Home Ministry

Pamela S. Hart, MDiv

At a Sunday morning worship service in a nursing home, I invited those attending to share with me their favorite verses from Scripture. I wrote each verse down on an index card as they were given to me. Later, as I looked over the cards, I was interested to find that every verse contributed came from the Psalms. The book of Psalms hold great meaning for people of faith. It is a trusted companion for a lifetime. Psalms are a reliable source of comfort and assurance throughout life and especially in the later years.

Why do the Psalms speak so clearly to the needs of humanity? The Psalms are the voice of humanity–our own common humanity–speaking to God of the joys and sorrows of life–the afflictions and the blessings–the despair and the elation of being alive and a part of the human family. The Psalms are not descriptions of life. They are life itself. While we must learn much of our information about aging from textbooks and life experience, we may also learn about aging by reading the Psalms. They get us in touch with the human experience over a long period of time. They include the voices of the elders of Israel. They speak of life as it is with no effort to hide or cover-up the afflictions of life. The Psalms speak with and for the afflicted and for

Pamela S. Hart is a Presbyterian pastor serving parishes and as a chaplain. She has also taught instrumental music. She received her Master of Divinity from St. Paul School of Theology.

[Haworth co-indexing entry note]: "The Psalms as a Resource for Nursing Home Ministry." Hart, Pamela S. Co-published simultaneously in *Journal of Religious Gerontology* (The Haworth Pastoral Press, an imprint of The Haworth Press, Inc.) Vol. 12, No. 2, 2001, pp. 61-68; and: *Religion and Aging: An Anthology of the Poppele Papers* (ed: Derrel R. Watkins) The Haworth Pastoral Press, an imprint of The Haworth Press, Inc., 2001, pp. 61-68. Single or multiple copies of this article are available for a fee from The Haworth Document Delivery Service [1-800-342-9678, 9:00 a.m. - 5:00 p.m. (EST). E-mail address: getinfo@haworthpressinc.com].

© 2001 by The Haworth Press, Inc. All rights reserved. *61* this reason are particularly helpful to the elderly in nursing homes as well as to chaplains and ministers and lay visitors who call on them. I read Psalm 38 to a ninety-five year old woman who is losing her eyesight, "My heart throbs, my strength fails me; and the light of my eyes–it also has gone from me." Without a hesitation, she said, "Well, I can identify with that!"

The Psalms are honest about life. They show life with all its ups and downs. They leave the rough edges and do not try to smooth over all of the flaws and imperfections of human existence. Moreover, they go straight to God for answers. They demand a response. God is expected to answer for the tribulation in this life and not merely watch over creation like a passive spectator.

Walter Brueggemann, in *Praying the Psalms*, sees in them three different states of being. He names these states orientation, disorientation, and new orientation. The state of orientation is a state of equilibrium. Everything about life is understandable and secure. Life is going well. This state is the one most people want to be in and try to be in whether or not the facts of life actually warrant it. As Brueggemann says:

> For the normal, conventional functioning of public life, the raw edges of disorientation and reorientation must be denied or suppressed for purposes of public equilibrium. As a result, our speech is dulled and mundane. Our passion has been stilled and is without imagination. And mostly the Holy One is not addressed, not because we dare not, but because God is far away and hardly seems important.[1]

He goes on to say that words of the Psalms do not reflect the common, everyday kind of conversation that makes life sound agreeable and pleasant. The Psalms are clearly quite different in their "tell it like it is" approach. In fact, Brueggemann feels that the Psalms cannot be prayed aright except by people struggling with the "primitive passions" of life and the "raw hurts" that come when life is turned upside down and everything goes from bad to worse. According to Brueggemann, the oriented life does not create great prayer. Only when life is threatened and disrupted do people become truly eloquent and passionate in their prayers to God.[2]

Recently, I talked with a woman about growing old. "I'm a rebellious one," she kept saying. "I want to know why God doesn't just take us. What good are we anyway?" She spoke with the passion of Psalm 13.

> How long, O LORD? Wilt thou forget me for ever? How long wilt thou hide thy face from me? How long must I bear pain in my soul, and have sorrow in my heart all the day? (Psalm 13: 1-2)

Most older people I have met keep their anger hidden inside. They cover it up with pious words of gratitude. They feel guilty shaking their fists at God. This woman can't keep it inside. She wants an answer. She wants to know "Why? How long?" Unknowingly, she stands with the Psalmist who seethes with anger and hurt and bursts out in furor to the High and Holy God.

> Out of the depths I cry to thee, O LORD! LORD, hear my voice! Let thy ears be attentive to the voice of my supplications! (Psalm 130: 1-2)

Brueggemann writes that the Psalms of disorientation help us through the agonies of life including all the losses that accompany it at any age. These Psalms help us die to old situations. They help us see the end to any further possibilities of returning to a former state. They help us get rid of "false hopes, pretense, and old lines of defense." They help us see truly that whatever has happened is final. "That is all over now."[3]

> I am weary with my moaning; every night I flood my bed with tears; I drench my couch with my weeping. My eye wastes away because of grief, it grows weak because of all my foes. (Psalm 6: 6-7)

The Psalms show that we do not have to hide our feelings about life. We do not have to deny the hurt we feel. The Psalms show that people can take everything that disturbs them to God and trust their problems to the Holy One.

New orientation always comes unexpectedly. In the darkest hours, God comes. God comes to people through gifts that touch people where they are hurting. Perhaps God comes in an act of kindness or through the gift of friendship.

> I waited patiently for the Lord; he inclined to me and heard my cry. He drew me up from the desolate pit, out of the miry bog,

and set my feet upon a rock, making my steps secure. He put a new song in my mouth, a song of praise to our God. Many will see and fear, and put their trust in the LORD. (Psalm 40: 1-4)

The Psalms portray the joys of life along with the sorrows of death. The Psalms call us to the realities of human existence. Before resurrection comes crucifixion. People suffer many deaths over a lifetime. The Psalms can assist the bereaved in their times of sorrow and heal the broken heart. The Psalms are a resource for healing. They are the voices of human beings who know and understand how chaotic life can be, yet confidently affirm that God does not abandon the living to their sorrow but delivers them out of the pit and redirects their lives.

My role as Chaplain gave me an opportunity to utilize the insights of Walter Brueggemann's book, *Praying The Psalms* and apply them to pastoral care, preaching, and Bible study. I categorized the Psalms according to the needs I saw in this setting. When I completed this process, I began to use these verses as prayers and devotionals in pastoral care situations. One woman I saw had no family or friends living close by. Her niece wrote to me and asked If I would visit her aunt since she lived so far away. The woman was bedridden. Her face was thin and drawn. Her hair was thick and gray and her forehead rough and worn. When I stood beside her bed, she said, "I hurt. I hurt. Oh, God. I hurt." I took her hand and began to say the Twenty-third Psalm. She started to say it with me. "Though I walk through the valley of the shadow of death, I shall fear no evil, for Thou art with me. Thy rod and thy staff they comfort me." We walked together through the "valley of the shadow of death." I was in that valley everyday. The Psalm was a comfort to me as well as the patient. I was not alone. Jesus said, "For where two or three are gathered in my name, there am I in the midst of them" (Matthew 18: 20).

Life is very difficult for many persons living in nursing homes. One woman's face always bore the strain of life. Her favorite Bible verse was "Cast thy burdens upon the Lord, and he shall sustain thee . . ." (Psalm 55: 22 KJV). She came regularly to chapel and to Bible study. She knew from the years she spent as a nurse that people who make the effort to get better improve much faster than those who refuse to try. It is an effort for her to keep trying for her hearing is poor and her strength is giving out. How much easier it would be to stay in her room and watch television. But she is in touch with the voice of the

Psalmist who assured her that no burden is too difficult for God to bear and so she "casts her burden on the Lord" and doesn't give up.

I soon discovered that I was not the only one giving pastoral care. Several of the residents made calls on the sick. They dropped by to bring the mail or read or visit. They comforted and reassured others by their presence and concern. They showed to the ones who were sick or disabled that God had not left them alone but comes to them through those who are moved by the love of Jesus Christ to give of themselves for others as Jesus gave of himself for the salvation of all. "If I were here on this floor, I surely would want someone to visit me," a resident said to me after I recognized her cheerful presence.

Many others, however, were caught in the pit. They live in *sheol*, that shadowy world of the dead where God is not to be found. They could not see how life had anything left to offer them. The losses had been too great. "This is no way to live," a person said to me. "I wish I'd never given up my home in Arkansas. I had to come here. My doctor insisted and so did my daughters. But I don't like it here and I wish I had never given up my home. This is no way to live."

Preaching from the Psalms offers a chance to speak to the unexpected and unhappy changes that come to everyone in life. One collection of sermons called *Sermons From the Psalms* by Clovis G. Chappell offers a splendid resource for developing sermons for nursing home patients. Chappell selects a very brief text and expounds on the meaning giving one illustration after another in a very energetic and uplifting manner. The sermon, "A Radiant Certainty," is based on the text of Psalm 56: 9. "This I know, that God is for me." The sermon has three main points. The Psalmist knows that God is. He knows that God cares. He knows that God is working on his behalf. Chappell's style must be heard in his own words:

> Finally, the psalmist discovered, not only that God cares, but that he is working on his behalf. He is seeking in every way within his power to bring him to his finest self and to his highest possibilities. This does not mean that his road was always made soft by a carpet of flowers. God did not coddle him and pamper him. He did not protect him from every rude wind. On the contrary, his road was at times heartbreakingly rough and rugged. He knew what it was to pass sleepless nights; he had an intimate and long acquaintance with tears. But he has become convinced that God

is working for his enrichment, not only in spite of all his difficulties, but also even through them. His tears are being conserved. They are being kissed into jewels. His loses are being transformed into glorious gains. Thus in the face of disappointment and sorrow he can still sing, 'God is for me.'[4]

The psalms preach! They speak with the human voice. What nursing home resident cannot attest that the road in life is at times "heartbreakingly rough and rugged?" Who among them has not had "sleepless nights," especially that first month after the day they moved in? Which one doesn't need to hear the radiant words, "This I know that God is for me.'

Chappell has another sermon entitled "Keeping Our Footing." It is based on Psalm 73: 2. "But as for me my feet were almost gone; my steps had well-nigh slipped." The sermon takes on all of the questions people ask when they stumble in life and fall down and feel like quitting. Using the Psalmist as the illustration of faith in the midst of tribulation is one of the strongest approaches to the difficult questions of life. Where are you God? Are you really there? Chappell handles these questions in this way:

> The other day I saw a mother going down the street with her little child. For a few steps the little fellow walked alone, but he came to where a crossing was to be made. He then reached up and the mother took his hand and he went forward without fear. 'So it has been in my case,' says the Psalmist. 'When the way grew rugged and treacherous and I was in danger of losing my footing, I reached up my hand. And when I did so I did not clutch the thin air. Instead, there was One who seized my hand and held it fast, and who steadied me and gave me guidance.'[5]

The more I study Chappell's sermons the more relevant the Psalms become as a source of spiritual nourishment in nursing home ministry. As soon as I read this sermon I thought of a resident who recently fell and broke her hip. I thought of the pain she suffered from the fall and the surgery that followed. I thought of the sorrow she felt when the minister of her church failed to visit her in the hospital until she was ready to go home. At least he came. But she had reason to expect more. Before her husband's retirement, he was Minister of Pastoral Care at that church!

Leslie Brandt in *Psalms Now* gives a contemporary rendering of Psalm 120 giving expression to what this woman felt as she waited for her pastor to come:

> I am distressed, O Lord, by the attitudes and actions of those who claim to honor your name and to live within Your presence. They don't really listen to Your Word. They appear to be following some other god or are simply taking the path of least resistance.[6]

The Psalms reach. The Psalms preach. And the Psalms teach. Bible study in small groups gives people a chance to discuss the feelings of the Psalmist and to share their own. I have found it to be true, as Brueggemann indicates, that people prefer the appearance of faith. They are hesitant to open themselves to others and admit they have doubts or fears. They are even more hesitant to admit anger. Nevertheless, a discussion of the lament Psalms or Psalms of disorientation gives people permission to be honest with God and may have a positive effect on their private devotions.

In my presentation of the Psalms, I followed Brueggemann's organizational pattern but changed the terms to Psalms of Praise, Psalms of Lament, and Psalms of Renewal. In his second book, *The Message of the Psalms*, Brueggemann writes that the Psalms of Praise were written for liturgical purposes and for supporting the status quo. They did not reflect the real life experiences of many people.[7] The Psalms of Lament, however, were true to life and expressed the tension people felt when life was at its worst. The Psalms of Renewal were the result of new insight and direction received during times of stress and spoke with a confidence that knew adversity but no longer despair. During our class, a woman shared her thoughts with us, "When I pray to God, I may not get an answer right away, but if I wait, the answer comes." In these Psalms, trust in God is born anew. Life is transformed.

The study of the Psalms as a resource in nursing home ministry continues to influence how I minister to older persons generally. The more knowledge I have of the Psalms, the more ways I find to utilize them in my everyday ministry. Moreover, I will continue to study them for my own benefit as well. They are a rich source of experience giving much insight into the human condition. The Psalms give me a deeper understanding of life and make me realize that the human cries of anguish come out of an intolerable life situation. It is a reminder to me that life is not forever in a state of equilibrium but will certainly change (and possibly for the worse).

This study, I believe, has shown that the Psalms are an essential resource for nursing home ministry. Knowledge of the Psalms is beneficial not only to the residents and patients, but also to ministers and chaplains. Here, in this setting, is a high concentration of people who are experiencing many of the same feelings of anguish and forsakenness that the Psalmist describes. The Psalms can prepare the minister or chaplain to be with those in sorrow, and they can provide hope for all that God does indeed make his presence known to them even in times of darkness, and God will not leave them in the pit but will take them to a safe and secure place where they can find protection and care and loving kindness.

The more familiar the Psalms become to the minister or chaplain the more possibilities for their use will present themselves. I would like the Psalms to become so much a part of my prayer life and teaching that I do not even realize I am using them.

As the voice of humanity speaking to God, the Psalms hold an honored place among our Sacred Writings. They are the voice of ancient Israel and the voice of every generation of the Christian community in dialogue with God. The limitations on the usefulness of the Psalms as a resource will be the result of their importance in the view of the chaplain or minister working in that facility rather than with the Psalms themselves. Integrating the Psalms into the life of a nursing home should be a joyous and meaningful and challenging task for a creative person interested in the spiritual nourishment of the elderly. The Psalms are a timeless treasure and a blessing to nursing home ministry.

NOTES

1. Brueggemann, Walter, *Praying the Psalms*. Winona: Christian Brothers Publishing Company, 1982, p. 19.

2. Ibid., p. 20.

3. Ibid., p. 30.

4. Chappell, Clovis B., *Sermons From the Psalms*. Nashville: Cokesbury Press, 1931, p. 98.

5. Ibid., p. 88.

6. Brandt, Leslie F., *Psalms Now*. St. Louis: Concordia Publishing Company, 1973, p. 190.

7. Brueggemann, Walter, *The Message of the Psalms*. Minneapolis: Augsburg Publishing Company, 1984, p. 26.

Communication with Older Persons: Part I– Looking Within

Robert E. Buxbaum, DMin, ACSW

Two groups with whom most adults have difficulty communicating are teenagers and the elderly. Adults who are perfectly comfortable with and adept at communicating with others often find themselves uncomfortable, anxious and even angry when relating to these two groups. Both adolescents and the aged seem to demand of us special effort and understanding if we are to reach them. Perhaps, on some level, they intentionally complicate the communication process forcing us to prove we care enough to unravel the puzzle before they become vulnerable. They stand as chronological bookends on either side of the stages of adulthood most coveted and dreaded by our society. One is not yet within the mainstream of adult society, the other is inexorably slipping beyond. Each needs affirmation, assurance that they are loved, cared for, valued. Both are sensitive to any sign of rejection, any attempt to deal with them involving less than complete honesty, any response that does not take them seriously. When treated poorly, they respond with anger, withdrawal, oppositional behavior and regression.

Robert E. Buxbaum (deceased) was the Director of Robert E. Buxbaum and Associates in San Antonio, Texas, a group of individual, marital, family and group therapists, at the time of the writing of this article. He was a minister in the Presbyterian Church (U.S.A.), Adjunct Faculty at McCormick Theological Seminary and the Oblate School of Theology.

[Haworth co-indexing entry note]: "Communication with Older Persons: Part I-Looking Within." Buxbaum, Robert E. Co-published simultaneously in *Journal of Religious Gerontology* (The Haworth Pastoral Press, an imprint of The Haworth Press, Inc.) Vol. 12, No. 2, 2001, pp. 69-77; and: *Religion and Aging: An Anthology of the Poppele Papers* (ed: Derrel R. Watkins) The Haworth Pastoral Press, an imprint of The Haworth Press, Inc., 2001, pp. 69-77. Single or multiple copies of this article are available for a fee from The Haworth Document Delivery Service [1-800-342-9678, 9:00 a.m. - 5:00 p.m. (EST). E-mail address: getinfo@haworthpressinc.com].

© 2001 by The Haworth Press, Inc. All rights reserved.

While the purpose of this essay is to focus on communication with the aged, their kinship with adolescents reminds us they are not completely unique in the ages of humanity. Just as with young persons, certain characteristics of the aged as a population group require our attention if we are to communicate effectively with them. Exploring these features and incorporating them into the traditional guidelines for effective communications can facilitate the development of meaningful relationships with older persons. But, prior to accommodating for these distinctions, we need to face the reality that two of the most prominent barriers to meaningful communication with older persons lie within ourselves.

LOOKING WITHIN

Communicating with older persons is complicated by two obstacles which arise out of our own humanity: our finitude and our experiences with our families of origin. If we did not have to manage our feelings about our own death–to which aging is the gateway–our anxieties about parents and grandparents, communicating with aged persons would be relatively simple and joyful. The truth, however, is that relating to older persons arouses feelings with us that get in the way. They symbolize realities which stimulate forebodings of the future and awaken painful memories of the past. Thus, barriers within ourselves require our foremost attention. Only as we allow our own resistances to enter our conscious awareness can we be free to move beyond them. As with many significant communication problems, we must begin to search for the solution by looking within.

Relating to the elderly involves coming in contact with our own future. We are exposed to an intimacy with the process by which the life cycle draws to a close. We are confronted with the inescapable realization that we too shall grow old and die.

> Student Chaplain: "Is Mr. Andrews terminal?"
> Nurse: "Aren't we all?"

Most of us spend the greater part of our lives oblivious to this fact. When we involve ourselves with elderly persons, however, we discover that maintaining this delusion becomes extremely difficult. With that realization, our avoidance and denial dissolve and we expose the anxieties aroused by facing the stark reality of our limited existence. In order to re-establish emotional equilibrium, to regain control of our feelings, to bring anxiety within manageable limits, we often create distance–whether actual or perceived–between ourselves and those persons who have forced these painful realities upon us. Sometimes we find other mechanisms that provide the safety of structure. Nevertheless, our response to the elderly is not really hostile or uncaring, as it so often is interpreted. Our response is simply human; even though the result may be clumsy behavior that causes undue pain to others.

Many persons who work with the aged, or who are in some way their advocates, attempt to motivate caring by exacerbating feelings of guilt. They seem to believe that if they can make family, friends and community feel guilty enough, we will recognize the error in our ways, visit frequently, and exhibit concern. For brief periods of time this strategy may work. But guilt is never a positive motivator for permanent change. In fact, since those of us who avoid close contact with the elderly do so largely out of discomfort, guilt only increases our uneasiness and reinforces our desire to stay away. We must help each other understand WHY we behave in ways that even we dislike. In so doing we can provide support for behavioral change and increase the number of options from which we can choose.

The ways in which we attempt to cope with our anxieties are almost too painful to enumerate. Frequently we cannot bring ourselves to visit at all! Note how we tend to delay such visits and to welcome, with a quiet sign of relief, the "intrusion" of other, more important demands upon our time. Apprehension surrounds us as we approach the entrance to a hospital or nursing home. We tire quickly, find refuge in relating to the octogenarian as if he or she were a child, offer physical gifts rather than the gifts of time, attention and presence, and discourage conversation about emotions, especially fear and grief.

> Mother: I'm grateful for all I have but I guess an old person like me doesn't have much to look forward to . . .

> Son: Now, mom, don't talk like that. You know that we come to visit as often as we can. . .

These reactions occur not because we are callous or uncaring but because, as humans, we are prone to defend ourselves against the anxiety engendered by this confrontation with feelings remarkably similar to our own.

As visitors to hospitals or nursing homes we are sometimes shocked by what we see as staff members relate to patients or residents. Couldn't that attendant have taken just a moment more to respond to the patient who cries out for Kleenex? Shouldn't that nurse have seen to it that someone called the person's family to tell them of his or her needs? Is a telephone conversation an adequate way for the physician to provide medical care? Some nursing home personnel are cold, uncaring, even cruel. But many are warm, tender, and considerate. In essence, they, too, are simply human beings. Their jobs, even their professional training, may not have prepared them to deal with their own anxieties.

Many times we project our own need to be distant upon those who care for the aged. We attempt to handle our guilt by expressing anger toward them.

> Daughter: I just get furious when I get here and see that they haven't given mother her bath yet. Lord only knows how she gets neglected when I'm not able to come by and check up. We pay a lot of money. . .

> Social Worker: You feel badly that you can't give your mother as much attention as you might like. The feeling that she *might* be neglected really hurts. . . .

Caregivers might be envisioned as lightening rods that attract the anger born of our own guilt. Many persons providing care for the elderly must contend not just with their own feelings about aging, but also with the resentment and anger of friends and relatives. Since their jobs often depend upon whatever goodwill they can elicit from these persons, they suppress their desire to retaliate and instead express anger and hostility toward their work. The burnout rate among caregivers for the aged may, in part, be attributed to being caught in this bind.

We expect a lot from those who care for the aged. More than we, ourselves, can provide. We tend to lose sight of the fact that their jobs have high stress levels and they, too, are struggling to overcome barriers within themselves. The regularity of their contact with people who remind them of their own aging and death often causes them to cultivate tremendous defenses against their anxieties. To some extent professionalism provides them with rituals and procedures which create distance, but the assumption that their training releases them from anxiety is quite erroneous. In fact, often the reverse is true. Behavior that seems abrupt, harsh, or uncaring usually is motivated by their anxiety over becoming too deeply enveloped in the plight of those for whom they care.

Since anxiety about aging and death is part of the human condition, we must admit to the ways in which we are influenced by such emotions. Underneath, we do not seek to avoid the aged but our own fears about aging. Note the curious fact: the aged seldom seem to have difficulty in visiting each other. Theoretically, should not they, for whom death is imminent, experience even higher anxiety levels and increased desire for avoidance? The logic of such a hypothesis is contradicted by the reality that the normal movement of the life cycle invites utilization of resources appropriate to our needs. If things have proceeded well by the time we enter the last phase of the life cycle, we will have amassed ego strength born of accomplishment, satisfaction and perspective which provides us with numerous coping mechanisms. The losses, physical limitation, diseases and disabilities of old age may not only bring on death, but may also increase our receptivity to it.

> You know," said the eighty-four year old man who was facing the possibility of surgery, it isn't that I fear death. I've had a long and good life. What I fear is that I might die before my wife. Who would visit her in the nursing home? Who would see that she was taken care of? Once she dies, death would not be unwelcome.

Perhaps such an outlook suggests that younger persons might benefit by trying to view the world of the aged through the eyes of the aged. In classes on counseling older persons, students have found writing fantasies of their retirement years and their own deaths to be very helpful. By imaging themselves fifty or sixty years ahead, they gain new and different insight into what it means to be old and to die. Coming close to the actual experiences of aging and death through such fantasies allows them to be less hesitant about initiating relationships with older persons. Discovering that, with age many people become less anxious and more accepting of death, helps them to cope better with their own anxieties.

The second inner barrier to communicating with older persons is the extent to which they remind us of our parents and grandparents and reactivate unresolved conflicts. Perhaps this can be understood best by reviewing some of the ways our relationships with each of these generations affect our current efforts to communicate with the elderly.

Keeping boundary lines clear, keeping identities separate, is often a difficult task. When we deal with older persons, we may be reminded of situations we have encountered with our own parents and this remembrance may cloud our judgement.

> Son: When you saw mother getting increasingly depressed after dad died, why didn't you refer her to a therapist?

> Physician: When *my* father died and mother became depressed, I referred her to a psychiatrist. He only made matters worse.

We may experience some older individuals as possessing qualities we have desired in our parents. Or, they may remind us of our parents' negative qualities. In essence, we may find ourselves being angry, judgmental and rejecting toward the aged persons before us without being fully aware of why we are reacting in such a manner.

Some of us have painful recollections of relationships with our parents and the problems between us rarely disappear with age. We find better ways of coping with them, but they are likely to remind us and may even be aggravated by the subtle shifts in roles and in our needs.

> My father calls me up all the time now that mother is becoming senile. He cries and complains. He wants me to listen to his problems, to understand his feelings! He never listened to me! All those years that I wanted to be able to talk with him and now. . . .

Perhaps, we see our parents relating to our own children in ways that spark painful memories and anger.

> It makes me furious to see her treating my kids the same way she treated me! You'd think by now she would have learned. Well, I couldn't say anything when she did that to me, but now . . . .

Either consciously or unconsciously older persons may remind us of our parents and unearth feelings we thought were relegated to the past. If we are to minimize the effect of these barriers, we must be aware of such unresolved feelings and, whenever possible, work on concluding them.

Also, relationships with our grandparents can affect the way we communicate with older persons. For example, often, when in conflict with parents, we turn to grandparents for emotional satisfaction and positive role models. In fact, we may tend to idealize them.

> Whenever I couldn't get along with my parents, I turned to grandma. When my parents would get angry at me for not eating my vegetable, she'd eat them for me. . . It's only been recently, in the last few weeks, that I've come to realize that I've been looking for someone to save me from unpleasant situations ever since!

Some of us carry into our relationships with the elderly the desire to see them as we need them to be. We are more prone to sentimentalize our view of grandparents than parents. Grandparents have the advantage of relating to their grandchildren without the stress of responsibility shouldered by parents. Overindulgent, or worldly wise, philosophical grandparents are loved easily by children. Unfortunately, we often expect the older persons we deal with to confirm our fond reflections, and when they do not, we feel betrayed.

Unlike the idealized image, some grandparents are cold, rejecting, disinterested, afraid, jealous, and too caught up in their own anxieties and unresolved emotional needs to be able to respond appropriately. They may be unable to give the kind of warmth, support and care their grandchildren desire. As humans, they, too, have problems. They need affirmation and may seek it inappropriately from their grandchildren; expecting more than the grandchildren have the resources to give.

In short, experiences with our own grandparents–whether rewarding or painful–can have a profound affect on our relationships with older persons. Therefore, it is important to look at those experiences honestly. Only then can we view the person before us as a unique individual rather than a reflection of our own perceptions.

Another side of this issue is worthy of note. Relationships with our family of origin may also provide the motivation for initiating relationships with older persons. If intimate involvement in the lives of our parents and grandparents has been a rewarding experience, relating to other older persons may seem extremely appealing. On the other hand, if may be unresolved negative emotions or certain emotional deprivations which provoke us into seeking out the elderly. In short, the same agendas which distort our ability to respond appropriately to older persons may lead us to seek them out in the first place. However, the degree to which the motivation for developing relationships with the elderly is a negative factor depends largely on our awareness.

> I looked forward to introducing my father to the man who had become my mentor. My older colleague had taught me so much and was a close friend. It wasn't until I was introducing them and my father said, 'I'm glad to meet my competition,' that I realized how much my friend was the kind of person that I always wanted my father to be!

Anxieties about death and unresolved emotional issues with grandparents and parents may so distort our perceptions that they affect what we hear, how we respond, and even our incentive for initiating relationships. Clearly, the process of communicating with older persons is so intertwined with basic life and family of origin issues that those who want to improve their skills must first become more aware of themselves. The question often arises as to whether such issues must be settled on our own or with help from a third party. In some situations, a professional therapist can assist by helping to identify, understand, and hopefully alleviate our fears and concerns. In fact, the insight and growth derived from a personal therapeutic experience may encourage us to work out our conflicts with parents and grandparents directly. Thus, a professional helping person, such as a counselor, may be useful in clarifying issues and feelings so they can be discussed more openly with the persons actually involved in the problem(s).

Many children believe that their parents are too old to change and therefore, attempts to address longstanding issues are inevitably fruitless. True, some older persons are less prone to make changes than are younger persons. Some may be unable to make any significant changes at all. However, older persons, even our parents, are frequently more ready to talk about the realities of their life experiences than we realize. As a psychotherapist, family counselor, and an ordained minister who relates to a variety of older persons, I frequently am impressed by their courage in making realistic evaluations of their lives. Often, they experience welcome relief in being able to talk freely and honestly about their feelings. In fact, sometimes they are more ready to change than their children and grandchildren are prepared to accept. Almost always, at least on some level, older persons are acutely aware of the problem everyone is avoiding and the silence makes them feel isolated and unloved. Having talking about it, however, having faced even the most painful of realities, the distance between their children and themselves begins to dissolve. Both are now free to build a closer, more meaningful relationship.

Perspectives on Aging:
Jewish, Roman Catholic, Protestant

Lindsey P. Pherigo, PhD

This paper will attempt to describe some of the religious, theological, and biblical aspects of aging, as understood by Judaism, Roman Catholicism, and Protestantism, in their traditional forms. By traditional forms, I mean Talmudic Judaism, pre-Vatican II Roman Catholicism, and the Protestantism rooted in the Lutheran and Reformed traditions. I am quite aware that there are a healthy variety of positions within each of these traditions, but this variety does not obliterate some basic shapes of each as they have expressed themselves in history.

I am also aware that there are cross currents of theology that find powerful representatives in all three traditions, from the "fundamentalists," on one extreme, to "process theologians" on the other–with "charismatics" and "liberals" somewhere along the continuum between. Time and space alone, to say nothing of the need for a focus, preclude my taking all these cross currents into our discussion. It will be sufficient now to deal with the three great Western expressions of religion in their mainstream, more-or-less orthodox, forms.

With this plan, all three traditions will perhaps feel poorly represented. Judaism, for example, will respond with a protest from the Reform group–or even from the Conservative–that they aren't fully

Lindsey P. Pherigo is Professor Emeritus of New Testament and Early Church History at Saint Paul School of Theology, Kansas City, Missouri. He holds a PhD in Church History from Boston University. He is an ordained United Methodist minister.

[Haworth co-indexing entry note]: "Perspectives on Aging: Jewish, Roman Catholic, Protestant." Pherigo, Lindsey P. Co-published simultaneously in *Journal of Religious Gerontology* (The Haworth Pastoral Press, an imprint of The Haworth Press, Inc.) Vol. 12, No. 2, 2001, pp. 79-87; and: *Religion and Aging: An Anthology of the Poppele Papers* (ed: Derrel R. Watkins) The Haworth Pastoral Press, an imprint of The Haworth Press, Inc., 2001, pp. 79-87. Single or multiple copies of this article are available for a fee from The Haworth Document Delivery Service [1-800-342-9678, 9:00 a.m. - 5:00 p.m. (EST). E-mail address: getinfo@haworthpressinc.com].

© 2001 by The Haworth Press, Inc. All rights reserved.

included. Roman Catholics will object that nothing is the same since Vatican II, and to exclude it is to deal with "the way it was." Protestants of the Radical Wing of the Reformation (Baptists, Mennonites, Quakers, Congregationalists, etc.) or of the Church of England's quasi-Catholicism, or of the nineteenth century American evangelical revival movements (Adventists, Latter Day Saints, Pentecostals), or of the neo-Gnostic resurgents (Christian Science, Unity)–all will feel excluded, and rightly so. But focus is needed, and it is here that we can make a beginning.

In Judaism, the starting point is the doctrine of creation. Human beings were created "in the image of God" and God declared the creation of humans as "very good." From this starting point the rabbis in the period that formulated historical Judaism as it is known in the Common Era explained aging as a positive aspect of life. Aging was part of the divine plan, part of God's gift of life. The Reform Prayerbook is faithful to traditional Judaism when it includes the insight:

> When tears dim our vision and grief clouds our understanding, we often lose sight of His eternal plan. Yet we know that life and death, growth and decay, all reveal His purpose.[1]

Because of this positive orientation, Judaism has venerated the old persons within it and accorded them a high degree of respect. They are accorded both "honor" (*kibbud*) and reverence (*morah*). Honoring means performing positive acts of service. Reverencing means avoiding any disrespectful acts. The child-parent relationship epitomized by the commandment "Honor they father and thy mother" is a relationship that is applicable throughout life.

When the Jewish aged suffer physical and/or mental deterioration, the question of filial honor and reverence comes sharply into question. In the Talmud the question is put this way, "How far does the honor of parents extend?" (Kiddushim 31a). One strand of rabbinic teaching set no limits on the honor due parents, no matter how senile. Thus Rabbi Dimi reported that once Dama ben Netinah "was seated among the great men of Rome, dressed in a silken garment, when his mother came and tore the garment from him, slapped him on the head, and spat in his face–but he did not shame her" (ibid). Rabbi Eliezer taught that even if the father throws the wallet of the son into the sea, the son still show *morah* (reverence) and does not shame him. Maimonides, in the twelfth century, supports this tradition and utilizes these Talmudic illustrations to conclude:

> How far must one go to honor one's father and mother? Even if they took his wallet full of gold pieces and threw it into the sea before his very eyes, he must not shame them, show pain before them, or display anger to them; but he must accept the decree of scripture and keep his silence. And how far must one go in his reverence? Even if he is dressed in precious clothes and is sitting in an honored place before many people and his parents come and tear off his clothes, hitting him in the head and spitting in his face, he may not shame them, but he must keep silent, and be in awe and fear of the King of Kings who commanded him thus. (Mamrim 6: 7)

Maimonides, however, did establish a different responsibility in dealing with a parent who is mentally disturbed.

> If one's father or mother should become mentally disordered, he should try to treat them as their mental state demands, until they are pitied by God. But if he finds he cannot endure the situation because of their extreme madness, let him leave and go away, deputing others to care for them properly. (Mamrim 6: 10)

Talmudic scholars suggest that this judgment of Maimonides stems from this Talmudic story: "Rabbi Assi had an aged mother. Said she to him, 'I want ornaments.' So he made them for her. 'I want a husband as handsome as you.' Thereupon he left her [in Babylon] and went to Palestine" (Kiddushim 31b). Note that even in this case, the care of the aged parent is still the responsibility of the son. The conclusion? "Abnormal" parental behavior must be patiently borne, but the care of a mentally deranged parent can be delegated to others. The ever-present ambiguity is the distinction between "abnormal" and "mentally deranged": how does one determine which is the case?

How far is it legitimate to transfer standards for aged parents to aged persons in general? While caution is appropriate here, the principles transfer well. Aging increases one's status in Jewish circles, not only with one's children, but with the community as well. The Hebrew scriptures lay down as an imperative, "You shall rise up before the greyhaired and defer to one who is older" (Leviticus 19: 32). It was the elders (literally, the old ones) who ruled the synagogue. Rabbi Abraham Heschel contrasts this regard for the aged with the youth-oriented culture of modern America.

> More time and money are spent on the art of concealing the signs of old age than on the art of dealing with heart disease and cancer. You find more patients in the beauty parlor than in the hospital. We would rather be bald than grey. A white hair is an abomination. Being old is defeat, something of which to be ashamed . . . [2]

Officially, however, Judaism, both biblically and theologically, views old age as the proper completion of a divine plan. It believes that old age can be rich and productive. It holds Moses as an ideal, who "was a hundred and twenty years old when he died; his eye was not dim, nor his natural forces abated" (Deut. 34: 7). Therefore, according to the divine plan, the Psalmist summarizes it well by saying

> We bring our years to an end as a tale that is told. The days of our years are threescore years and ten, or even by reason of strength fourscore years. . . . So teach us to number our days that we may get us a heart of wisdom. (Psalm 90: 10-12)

ROMAN CATHOLIC

Although Christianity adopted the Hebrew scriptures as its "Old Testament," and thereby preserved within its canon the *Imago dei* concept of the creation of humankind, it effectively nullified this with its doctrine of the Fall and subsequent depravity of humans. Instead of a foundational doctrine rooted in the powers of God the Creator, Christianity took its start from a negative estimate of the human condition that contributed strongly to the separation of Church and synagogue. "The Fall" caused the powers of sin and death to enslave the whole race (in the Pauline phraseology). Or, "the god of this world" has blinded the whole race to the reality of the true God (in Johannine phraseology). Whether enslaved by sin or by ignorance, all humans were in bondage and needed rescue.

In this Christian understanding death was allied with sin and the evil aspects of the universe. Death is the final enemy, overcome for us by the victory of Jesus in his resurrection. From this perspective, therefore, Christianity tended to view aging as movement toward death. It was a negative attitude. The infirmities of old age were its characteristic features.

Consequently, the respect and veneration of old age typical of Judaism is seldom found in classical forms of Latin Christianity. A Roman Catholic pamphlet addressed to the Catholics of San Antonio, Texas–dated April 10, 1978–is shockingly representative of this attitude. It is entitled "Catholic Lay Ministry to the Sick and the Aged." In it the *total* treatment of the aged is in the context of the sick. Nowhere is there any attention paid to the aged who are well and fully functional. Further illustrating the Roman Catholic tendency to be negative about aging is the way the elderly are usually in the custodial care of nuns who are nurses, and priests as they visit the sick. The lay movement to employ and vitalize the functional elderly has only very recently moved into Catholic circles.

Catholicism has often taught a general view of the meaning of life that has contributed to this negative approach. The function of life is to prepare oneself for the next life. Life is a discipline. Its hardships are character-developing experiences. Born as we are, in original sin, we need the Grace of God from start to finish. These "graces" were institutionalized in the sacraments, which functioned not only at each major lifephase, but especially in a regular on-going way through the Holy Eucharist as the Mass. Christians are pilgrims in a foreign land, on the way to "the City of God," to use St. Augustine's famous book-title. In this context, aging is mostly the last stage of this woeful pilgrim journey. It is easy to equate its special infirmities with illness, even when they are not. Death is the final end of life's miseries, and in this sense is sometimes welcomed by the Catholic faithful both as the end of a pilgrim journey in a strange hostile world and as the doorway to the new life with God. The poignant expression in Jesus Ben Sirach:

O death, how welcome is
your sentence
to one who is in need and is
failing in strength.
Very old and distracted
over everything.(41: 2, R.S.V.)

is essentially Catholic in spirit, in direct contrast to the Jewish spirit of the following verse:

Do not fear the sentence of death
Remember your former days and
The end of life.
This is the decree from the Lord
For all flesh
And how can you reject the
Good pleasure of the Most High? (R.S.V.)

PROTESTANT

Now, what about the Protestant view of aging? Strong in both the Lutheran and Reformed mainstream of classical Protestantism is the doctrine of election. It is understood as a necessary corollary of God's absolute sovereignty. Whereas election in Judaism primarily refers to the people as a whole, in Protestantism it is largely an individual matter. The most influential statement arose in Calvinism and was expressed as predestination.

When Calvinism is confronted with the all-important personal question, "How do I know if I'm one of the elect?" it answers, "By the life you lead." If you are truly one of the elect your life will be an expression of the grace of God within you. As we are by now very aware, this theology became the mainspring of Protestant industry, on a personal level, and a major root of modern capitalist society. Protestants don't work hard in order to be saved; they work hard to convince themselves (and others) that they are saved.

This Protestant doctrine has been a major influence in shaping Western society. The Catholic Henri Nouwen put his finger on the essential Protestant attitude toward aging when he noted that old people "become victims of a society which identifies their humanity with their productivity. . . ."[3] The society to which he refers (American) is a Protestant society, in which worth is established (proven) through productivity. Aging inevitably involves retirement. Retirement means no more work. No work, no value. It's a simple equation. Protestants tend to discard old people as no longer of any worth.

What is even more serious is that the discarded old have themselves "bought into" our society's Protestant value-system. Therefore they *feel* worthless and of no use. This feeling of worthlessness is very destructive of the actual values in the elderly, and sometimes multiplies infirmities and hastens death. The Psalmist has captured this well:

Those who see me in the street
Hurry past me
I am forgotten, as good as dead
In their hearts, something discarded.
(Psalm31: 11b-12; JB)

The Protestant work-ethic, as this is commonly called, places the center of one's value in one's work–what one produces. This is why, in our society, we are so interested in what a person does for a living. To know someone requires knowing what she or he does, for without that, the essential value of the person remains open. Protestantism values most highly the productive years; everything before that is preparation; everything after that is rest.

Protestants join Catholics in a common attitude of paternalism toward the aged, but for different reasons. Whereas the Catholic cares for the aged as infirmary patients, the Protestant cares for them as people who have outlived their usefulness. A certain element of condescension is more prevalent in Protestantism for the aged who are not independent; they tend to be regarded as a burden on society, and one that, if too visible, provokes guilt-feelings among the productive group. Protestants therefore have tended to isolate the elderly from society. In the more recent past this resulted in the creation of "Rest Homes" where they could be "kept." "Kept," meant "taken care of" but it also meant kept isolated from productive society.

In the still newer attitudes that are the results of gerontological research and findings, the emphasis includes rediscovering the values of the elderly–their wisdom, experience, and mature judgment. In this newer movement–surely a good thing in itself Protestants often unconsciously reapply their work-ethic that is the primary root of the condition of the aged. Making them useful again, in new ways, restores their value to society. The cycle starts all over; one's essential value resides in what one can do, in how useful a person is, in how well one can prove worth by productivity.

An alternative theological approach would critique this and propose that old persons be regarded as intrinsically, not instrumentally, valuable. It is noteworthy that old persons who are wealthy are not regarded as useless in our capitalist society. Their money makes them still productive and even powerful. Along with this acknowledgment is the common Protestant admiration for old people who are independent and self sufficient. This admiration is theologically grounded in the way their former productivity was good enough to provide well for their own non-productive period. They have doubly demonstrated their election.

Some modern movements have interacted with these theological perspectives, effectively challenging all three. Among these are evolution, historicism, and modern psychology.

If evolution correctly accounts for human origins, we humans are a biological becoming, and are perhaps still becoming. Our present stage is not a terminal stage, and all forms in the total process of becoming are only relatively valid. Their relative validity is simply their success in the experimental factors that account for change. Where now is the *Imago-dei* of the Jewish conception of a human being? What does that do to the meaning of life as a whole, and to the last stages in particular? This is not just a challenge to the Jewish perspective on human aging, but to the Christian also, because even in Christianity the present condition of sin, slavery, or ignorance is temporary; the original condition of the human race, personified in the Adam and Eve story, is also the eventual future of the race or at least of those who are "saved." A developing concept may be congenial with radical theologies like Process Theology, with its Jewish, Catholic, and Protestant representatives, but it certainly questions all three in their traditional garments.

Historicism has insisted that we are the continuous product of our own history with its man-made cultures. These cultures are each different from the others, and each is constantly changing anyway. These artificial constructs impose their values on us, and finally everything becomes relative. The biblical or theological constructs are not seen as absolutes, and "pluralism" is the order of the day. All ethical systems are thus profoundly challenged, including those that govern our perspectives on aging. Why is it "wrong" to exterminate the elderly, as some cultures do?

Modern psychology has debased the human animal most of all. The *Imago-dei* is now gone completely, and in its place are the depths of the subconscious. No longer do we take as our standard the God-image we used to believe in, but find our true nature and meaning in the lower realities that our higher nature hides and obscures. Nevertheless it is this lower nature that is the real self and it controls the rest. The human condition in Jewish perspective was on the right track with its slavery to sin doctrine, but now the condition of original sin has the stage to itself, with no contrasting and correcting *Imago-dei* in the wings. The basement has all the control panels.

The struggle now turns on a different axis. Those caught up in, and persuaded by, evolution, historicism, and modern psychology–whether Jew, Catholic, or Protestant–have entered on a new and different quest. It is the quest to achieve full humanity. "To become fully human" is the watch word of these questers. To become divine is hopeless mythology, "to become partakers of the divine nature" (2 Peter 1: 4) is an idle dream; it is hard enough to become fully human. Jews and Christians do this in different ways. I hear Jews saying this, but I don't know how they get there theologically. Christians do it by idealizing Jesus as the only fully human being we've had, and setting him us as our model.

The Lutheran Rudolf Bultmann claimed that in Jesus the possibilities of human existence were fully realized; he alone can make it possible for us to realize our fullest possibilities. Beyond that we cannot go. The Catholic John McKenzie proposed a Jesus who is "the standard by which the living and the dead are judged as valid human beings."[4]

The Lutheran and the Catholic just cited are both theologians without "Imprimatur." This modern "unorthodox" approach takes its own view of aging. It concentrates on the dignity and "humanity" all persons deserve. It holds high any program that furthers these traits in old age, and opposes most strongly "the monstrous indignities of the geriatric ward," not so much out of filial loyalty, honor, and reverence (the Jewish perspective), or out of pity and concern for the infirm and ailing (the Roman Catholic perspective), but on theological grounds that traditionalists regard as heretical, and heretical primarily because they are new and different.

NOTES

1. *Union Prayer Book*, (Central Conference on American Rabbis, vol. I, 1940) 73.

2. Heschel, Abrahana J. 1961. Unpublished paper delivered at the 1961 White House Conference on Aging, Washington, D.C.

3. Nouwen, Henri. 1974. Aging. New York: Doubleday.

4. McKenzie, John. 1980. *The New Testament Without Illusion*. Crossroad Publishing Co., pp. 28-29.

Three Approaches
to the Mystery of Suffering:
Frankl, Gray and Kushner

Leo E. Missinne, PhD

Many books and articles are written about suffering and the meaning of suffering. Some authors publish their story to alleviate their own pain, while others do so to help people cope with particular problems. Some look for answers to the universal question, "Is there some meaning in suffering?"

Suffering is very personal. It can be real or imagined. No two people suffer in the same degree from the same event. Situations that cause suffering may be the result of particular circumstances of a consequence of something we do to ourselves. Often, however, they are unexplainable. Why bad things happen to good people is a question all of us have asked, particularly when misfortune strikes or when we see how many good things happen to bad people.

Human existence has always been connected with suffering. Three persons: Viktor Frankl, Martin Gray, and Harold Kushner have coura-

Leo E. Missinne was Professor of Gerontology and a Graduate Fellow at the University of Nebraska at Omaha and Lincoln. He was also Visiting Professor in Gerontology at the University of Southern California, and is associated with the Center for the Study of Preretirement and Aging, National Catholic School for Social Service. Leo was ordained a Roman Catholic priest and belongs to the Society of Missionaries of Africa. He obtained his PhD in Educational Sciences at the University of Louvain in Belgium.

[Haworth co-indexing entry note]: "Three Approaches to the Mystery of Suffering: Frankl, Gray and Kushner." Missinne, Leo E. Co-published simultaneously in *Journal of Religious Gerontology* (The Haworth Pastoral Press, an imprint of The Haworth Press, Inc.) Vol. 12, No. 2, 2001, pp. 89-97; and: *Religion and Aging: An Anthology of the Poppele Papers* (ed: Derrel R. Watkins) The Haworth Pastoral Press, an imprint of The Haworth Press, Inc., 2001, pp. 89-97. Single or multiple copies of this article are available for a fee from The Haworth Document Delivery Service [1-800-342-9678, 9:00 a.m. - 5:00 p.m. (EST). E-mail address: getinfo@haworthpressinc.com].

© 2001 by The Haworth Press, Inc. All rights reserved.

89

geously faced it in ways that are an inspiration for others. Their stories give a unique and inspiring perspective.

VIKTOR FRANKL

Viktor Frankl, an emeritus professor of neurology and psychiatry at the University of Vienna, Austria, was exposed to suffering through his experiences in concentration camps during the Second World War. He is the founder of the school of logotherapy, which focuses on the meaning of existence and humankind's search for such meaning. Frankl was convinced that the need for meaning is a basic human need.

He was ready to publish the results of his research, his life's work, when he and his wife were taken to the concentration camp of Auschwitz. Their crime? They were Jewish. He spent three years as an inmate of different camps before he was released at the end of World War II. His wife, parents, brother, and two sisters perished in the Holocaust.

When Frankl entered Auschwitz, he hid his research manuscript in his clothing, but was forced to exchange his clothing for that of an inmate who had been sent to the gas chamber. In the pocket of his "new" clothes he found a copy of the main Jewish prayer, Shema Yisrail. This coincidence challenged him to *live* his thoughts instead of putting them on paper.

Frankl's life in Auschwitz was an example of love, faith, and hope in the midst of endless suffering. He was convinced that when confronted by suffering, one should replace the often asked question, "Why do I have to suffer?" with "Yes, it happened. Now what can I do?" This is only possible if one can find a reason to survive such circumstances.

Throughout this ordeal, Frankl chose to survive for his wife and family. While Frankl was performing forced labor he would think of his wife, who had been separated from him when they entered the camp. Although he did not know her fate, he related that "my mind clung to my wife's image, imagining it with an uncanny acuteness. I hear her answering me, saw her smile, her frank and encouraging look. Real or not, her look was more luminous than the sun which was beginning to rise."[1] It was during this time he realized that the salvation of people in this life is *though* love and *in* love.

By observing his own behavior as well as that of his fellow inmates, Frankl came to the conclusion that there is still another way to find meaning in life. Not only can it be found in creating a work, doing a deed, loving, or enjoying the goodness of another human being, it is also found in the way one stands up to suffering. He concludes that suffering will not have meaning unless it is necessary or unavoidable. A cancer that can be cured should not be endured by the patient as if it is his or her cross. That would be masochism rather than heroism.

Frankl believes that suffering can and will have meaning if it changes a person for the better. The way in which one accepts fate and the suffering it entails, gives opportunity for a deeper meaning to life, even under the most difficult circumstances. In a bitter fight for self-preservation, a person may forget about human dignity and become no more than an animal or an egoist. Each human being has a chance to make use of or forego the opportunities of attaining deep human values from a difficult situation.

A person's attitude toward suffering may be the only way to give meaning to his or her life. Frankl calls this an attitudinal value, and illustrates it by the following story:

> A colleague doctor turned to me because he could not come to terms with the loss of his wife, who had died two years before. His marriage had been very happy and he was not extremely depressed. I asked him quite simply: 'Tell me what would have happened if you had died first and your wife had survived you?' 'That would have been terrible,' he said, 'how my wife would have suffered.' 'Well you see,' I answered, 'your wife has been spared that, and it was you who had spared her, though of course, you must not pay by surviving and mourning her.' In that moment, his mourning had been given the meaning of sacrifice.[2]

How does one have a positive attitude toward suffering? Frankl believes that self-detachment will help a person create a positive attitude, and can be best achieved through a sense of humor. He observed that "by virtue of his capacity of self-transcendence, a person is capable of forgetting himself, giving himself, and reaching out for a meaning to his existence.[3] Surprisingly, Frankl found humor, even in Auschwitz. Humor is a weapon of the soul in the fight for self-preservation and transcendence. With humor one can rise above any kind of situation, even if only for a few seconds.

Faith in God will also help a person create a positive attitude. Despite all suffering, a deep faith in God, who is the ultimate meaning in life and the explanation of all that happens in life, will help a person cope with even the most difficult situation.

MARTIN GRAY

Martin Gray, as a child lived in a Warsaw ghetto during the Second World War, and from the age of fourteen was marked for extermination by the Germans. He was forced to wear an armband with a star, identifying him as a Jew. He chose, however, to fight the Nazis rather than passively accept his fate. He risked his life to smuggle food to his mother and brothers who were hidden behind a false cupboard in their apartment. When they were betrayed by a friend and herded aboard a train for the infamous concentration camp at Treblinka, he joined them in a rescue attempt. When he realized they had been murdered, he escaped and became active in the Polish resistance movement against the German army. He constantly envisioned the day when he would overcome the Nazis and avenge his family's deaths. When at last he marched victoriously into Berlin as an officer of the Russian army, he realized:

> My revenge was bitter. I could sense the fear around me, those lines of men and women waiting for a little water, and who suddenly froze, went silent, because I was passing. I too had lined up for a little water on the banks of the Vistula; I too had seen a uniformed stranger, who was absolute power and the new law, walk up to me. Old women in black, motionless, holding containers, men stooping over ruins, I know you. I know you, dead city, hungry and frightened, I know how to tell the victims from the butchers. They hit us first, and you let it happen, then they pushed you in front, like a shield. Today it's your turn. And we have butchers too.[4]

He recognized the suffering of the Germans because it mirrored his own suffering. The conflict between compassion and revenge raged inside him. Where would he find the solution to the conflict between good and evil, light and dark, peace and bitterness, and love and hate? Perhaps he was referring to this when he wrote, "Man has two roads always before him. And he must choose between them. Two roads between his eyes, two destinies. And he will travel so until the last second of his life."[5] While struggling with that conflict, he remembered the role of his mother. Her love gave him strength in his suffering. She was a very gentle, quiet person who had no need to speak, for all her acts were full of love. When he entered the first enemy town, ready to avenge the Germans, it was his mother's image that held him back.

When he and his fellow soldiers searched the town for the enemy, they found only the very old and the very young. Many of his fellow soldiers were completing the cycle of destruction begun by the Germans. They killed indiscriminately. While carrying out one of these searches, an incident occurred, which was a turning point in Gray's quest for meaning of life and of suffering.

> A child turned back toward the door of a cellar, his face was covered with tears. He wiped his nose with the back of his hand. He was waiting for someone to appear. An old woman came out, bent double by age–no doubt his grandmother. Reaching her hand to him she drew him to her, caressing his face as he buried himself in her black pleated skirt. This hand on a child's cheek; it was my mother with me. I shouted out an order. My comrades looked at me, shrugging their shoulders and spitting toward the inhabitants as they moved off. I was the last to leave, turning around to see this old woman and child, one against the other. My dead mother had saved me from the violent part of myself. Her gentleness and goodness had prevented me from letting it prevail over me.[6]

During all these difficult times, he lived for those he loved. The thought of his family gave him life. He knew that he could not succeed in avenging his family completely because they would never be restored to life. That is the failure of revenge. Death cannot be redeemed. Gray believed that only another life can efface death. His philosophy of life in the face of suffering, is perhaps best expressed in the following passage:

> . . . cold reason is not enough for man. It is merely the soil that must have water to germinate. The water is love, is others, is the hope and the belief that tomorrow, in each man and first of all

one's self, the fresh and beautiful will have sprung up. The certainty that man will be able to live in peace and joy, with himself and others. Any if suffering comes, and it will come since death will always be there, the hope that man will take this suffering into his hands and make it a fruit. To derive it the certainty that one must live a higher, better life, in fragile miracle which is life.[7]

HAROLD S. KUSHNER

Harold Kushner is a Jewish rabbi who had spent his adult life helping other people come closer to God. His son Aaron was born with progeria, the disease of rapid aging. He would never grow much beyond three feet in height, would have no hair on his head or body and would look like a little old man while he was still a child. He would die in his early teens. When the doctor gave him the diagnosis of his son, Kushner began to question his fate. He could not understand why that should happen to him? He recalls having a deep aching feeling of unfairness that did not make sense. He had always been a good person, as well as a good rabbi.

In order to help himself and others cope with this problem of unfairness, he decided to write a book.[8] Most of the literature he turned to for help in this time of suffering seemed to defend God's honor.

Where can a suffering human being go for help? Where can he or she turn for strength and hope? Kushner knew that he did not deserve punishment such as this from God, so he attempted to discover what God could mean to him after all.

Kushner believes that in this world, bad things do happen to good people, but it is not God who wills it. God is not controlling all the misery in the world. Sometimes things just happen. People have a free will and are often responsible for the circumstances. This approach will give one freedom. It will allow a person to recognize his or her basic goodness, and to feel that suffering is not a judgement or condemnation from God. One is free to be angry at what has happened and at life's unfairness, yet can feel compassion at seeing people suffer, because God teaches us both to be angry at injustices and to feel compassion for the afflicted. Instead of opposing God, we can believe that our indignation is God's anger at unfairness working through us.

When a person cries out, he or she is still on God's side, and God is still on his or hers. Kushner says:

> Christianity introduced the world to the idea of a God who suffers, along side the image of a God who creates and commands. Post biblical Judaism also occasionally spoke of a God who suffers, a God who weeps when He sees what some of His children are doing to others of His children. I don't know what it means for God to suffer. I don't believe that God is a person like me, with real eyes and real tearducts to cry, and real nerve endings to feel pain. But I would like to think that He is the source of my being able to feel sympathy and outrage, and that He and I are on the same side when we stand with the victim against those who would hurt him.[9]

Kushner's God is not only compassionate, He is a source of strength to those who suffer. Through prayer one can find strength and courage. Kushner observes that people in pain who pray often, discover that they have more strength and courage than they ever knew. Their prayers give them faith and courage unavailable before, because through prayer they come in contact with God's grace.

Those who suffer, not only need the strength found in prayer, but also need the support in talking to a caring friend. Kushner uses the example of Job. Job's friends did at least two things right. First, they had the courage to face him and to confront his sorrow and pain. Second, they listened to Job's complaints. According to the Bible, they sat with Job for several days, not saying anything, while Job poured out his grief and anger.

When we are questioned by someone as to why something bad has happened, it is important to agree that what has occurred is unfair. Along with caring and tenderness, this person needs help in keeping his or her mind and spirit strong in order to be able to think, plan, and make decisions in the future. To achieve this, Kushner advocates forgiveness and love. He believes that the best response to suffering is to forgive the world for not being perfect, to forgive God for not making a better world, and to reach out to the people around us and help them live in spite of all the pain and sorrow. "The ability to forgive and the ability to live are the weapons God has given us to enable us to live fully, bravely, and meaningfully in this less-than-perfect world." According to Kushner, our response to suffering can lead to either a positive or negative meaning.[10] It depends on us. Illnesses, accidents, and human tragedies are killing people, but they do not necessarily kill life, love, or faith. If the death and suffering of someone we love makes us bitter, jealous, against all religion, and incapable of happiness, we turn the person who died into someone responsible for our unhappiness and unbelief. In fact, we kill all life in ourselves because hatred is life unlived. If suffering and the death of someone encourages us to explore the limits of our capacity for strength, love and cheerfulness, and leads us to discover sources of consolation we never knew before, then we make the person who died into a witness for the affirmation of life.[11]

Kushner makes his son Aaron, who died shortly after his fourteenth birthday, a witness for the affirmation of life. He reveals, however, that it was not until he had gone beyond self-pity to the point of facing and accepting his son's death, that he was finally able to begin writing. His son's life was not in vain. It had a purpose. It would help others who were suffering.

Kushner realizes that telling people in his book how much it hurt will not do any good. His book must affirm life, love, and faith. It has to say that no one, neither Christ nor any other prophet, promises us a life free from pain and sorrow. Christ, however, promises that we will not be alone in our suffering. We can find ourselves in mystical union with Him, and through His example, survive life's tragedies and unfairness.

CONCLUSION

Suffering is not only a problem, it is a mystery. Mysteries are not solved by theories or intellectual approaches. When the Jewish people were looking for answers to the fundamental question of why people suffer, they turned to the book of Job. Job expressed the sentiments of a human in revolt, raising the ultimate protest against the injustices of life. Job argued with God, unable to understand how a just God could permit the suffering of an innocent. The example of Job is very typical. He expressed his feelings. For a long time Job was *with* God, then became *against* Him, but he could not be *without* Him. Not being able to live without God is the essence of what a religious person is all about.

Job was not Jewish. He was Gentile serving as an example for the

Jewish people. Three Jewish contemporary Jobs: Frankl, Gray, and Kushner, have been confronted with deep human suffering, and are now inspiring a Western Christian world. The roles seem to be reversed. They are a sign that suffering is a universal human phenomenon and not typical for a particular race, culture, or religion. Different philosophies and religions have proposed particular solutions for eliminating or minimizing suffering, but there is no one all-embracing answer for all people. Rather, there are many partial answers. Using the example of others, every human being must respond in his or her own way, inspired by the insights of his or her own faith.

These approaches to the problem of suffering, proposing different religious and philosophical attitudes, can be distressing to those who are searching for answers. Perhaps the best way to cope with suffering is to listen to those people, who in spite of many sufferings and in the midst of multiple questions, maintain a deep faith in God and peace of mind. Words never solve a problem.

NOTES

1. Victor Frankl, *Man's Search for Meaning* (New York: Pocket Books, 1963) 58-59.

2. Victor Frankl, *The Doctor and the Soul* (New York: Bantam Books, 1969), x.

3. Frankl, *Man's Search* . . . 106-107.

4. Martin Gray, *For Those I Loved* (Boston: Little, Brown & Company, 1972), 252.

5. Martin Gray, *A Book of Life* (New York: The Leabury Press, 1975), 201.

6. Ibid, 43-44.

7. Ibid, 209.

8. Harold S. Kushner, *When Bad Things Happen to Good People* (New York: Avon Books, 1983).

9. Ibid, 85.

10. Ibid, 147-148.

11. Ibid, 138.

In Wait for My Life:
Aging and Desert Spirituality

W. Paul Jones, PhD

Let me disclose the gifts reserved for age
To set a crown upon our lifetime's effort. . .
The end is where we start from.

–T.S. Eliot, "Little Gidding," *Four Quartets*

I remember being impressed years ago by Confucianism. Hardly any content remains to that memory, only the idea that life is composed of distinct periods that together make a person whole. No, there was a second idea. Life's crown is the final stage of spirituality, long formed by the maturing process of aging. It makes sense. One cannot expect from adolescent energy the quiet depth held in trust for later years, nor is childhood innocence to be ridiculed from the lofty heights of middle-age efficiency. "For everything there is a season" (Eccles. 3: 1). Thus each segment is to be drunk to its fullness, for its own sake, with none esteemed as higher than another. A person should savor one course, as it were, before going on to the next. Life so imaged becomes a pilgrimage, for in being shaped by a beginning and an end, living becomes imbued with plot.

The present Christian interest in story is a rediscovery of this narra-

W. Paul Jones is retired Professor of Theology at Saint Paul School of Theology, Kansas City, Missouri. He received his education at Yale University.

[Haworth co-indexing entry note]: "In Wait for My Life: Aging and Desert Spirituality." Jones, W. Paul. Co-published simultaneously in *Journal of Religious Gerontology* (The Haworth Pastoral Press, an imprint of The Haworth Press, Inc.) Vol. 12, No. 2, 2001, pp. 99-108; and: *Religion and Aging: An Anthology of the Poppele Papers* (ed: Derrel R. Watkins) The Haworth Pastoral Press, an imprint of The Haworth Press, Inc., 2001, pp. 99-108. Single or multiple copies of this article are available for a fee from The Haworth Document Delivery Service [1-800-342-9678, 9:00 a.m. - 5:00 p.m. (EST). E-mail address: getinfo@haworthpressinc.com].

© 2001 by The Haworth Press, Inc. All rights reserved.

tive nature of life. "We know who we are only when we can place ourselves–locate our stories within God's story."[1] Because "our lives are narrative dependent, . . . we are pilgrims on a journey."[2] Yet this truth discloses a basic dilemma: in modern society, such spiritual pilgrim aging is seriously undercut; for life's beginning and end as unique stages are tyrannized by the middle the years often called "productive."

COMPETITIVE FORMATION

Although our concern in this article is with the final years, the dilemma of both beginning and end is of a piece. Further back than children can remember, they are socialized to compete. My mother claimed that my father hung a ball glove above my crib. The child's hints of recognition, crawling, words each are parentally monitored for precociousness, endlessly compared with the offspring of neighbors and friends. Preschools institutionalize this dynamic, setting firmly in place the competitive dynamic of winner and loser as the foundation of modern education and life. Grades, assembly awards, making the varsity team, earning first chair. We are tracked early into positive or negative self-worth as established by "achievement."

So deep is this identification of "doing" with "meaning" that childhood as a distinct season of living is as threatened with extinction as an endangered species. The child's intrinsic awe and joy over life is devoured, rendered instrumental, as parents are pressured to provide a "head start" in their child's competition over others. Related is the institutionalization of childhood sports, as play for its own sake is poisoned, rendering it a "spring training" for life's deadly seriousness of winning by doing. Hovering over our class society is the "curve" of inevitable winners and losers. Once competition is burned into our motivational processes, the natural need for approval couples with the fear of being nothing until our innate aggressiveness is forged into an unquestioned, lifelong definition of "meaning."

Capitalism is the economic name for a society so conceived; individualism is the fate of the self so defined. When the Japanese House Speaker declared that Americans are "lazy," and their Prime Minister charged that we "lack a work ethic," they were attacking our very worth by faulting our performance according to those definitions of value by which we have always measured ourselves. Our knee-jerk defensiveness over these remarks is understandable.

However one may evaluate the wisdom of permitting such an understanding to characterize *any* period of life, there is solid reason for the Christian to question its centrality as model for the *whole* of life. Is such a measure of "success" compatible with a Christianity that insists that the first will be last, the rich will be sent empty away, the powerful will be pulled down, and the meek shall inherit the earth? The New Testament abounds with such "subversive" warnings, with implications ranging from economics to foreign policy: "Woe to you that are rich . . . that are full now . . . that laugh now . . . Woe to you, when all speak well of you" (Luke 6:24-26).

The gravitational pull of such environment upon the church is strong, justifying religion's value as means for acquiring the status and possessions most valued by our culture. Thus the race well run merges into the church's present obsession with growth as the religious "gross national product."

THE DESERT SPIRITUALITY

Throughout church history, this assimilation of Christianity into a culture's values has provoked, in time, prophetic reaction. One of the earliest and most profound of these reactions, called "desert spirituality," has served ever since as a potent model. It began under Constantine (312 C.E.), when accommodation of Christianity and culture became the policy of both state and church. Serious Christians entered the desert not to escape but to purify Christianity by doing battle in the wilderness which the powers and principalities called home.

My thesis is that society's aversion to the elderly is pushing them into a "desert." And while such rejection is often destructive, when viewed from the perspective of spirituality, aging can be restored to its unique integrity as the final stage of living. In so doing, the prophetic nature of Christianity can be modeled for all of us. The goal of such spirituality centers in the purifying of motive. If a person is religious in order to gain a larger reward in heaven than one could get by being irreligious on earth, Christians are little different from the Mafia. Both are trying to "make it" big–the only real difference being the stadium chosen for competing.

The desert *ascesis*, then, is indispensable for the conversion of motive. Put bluntly, *to become a Christian, a person must become a failure intentionally.*[3] Christianity is for losers, so much so that "winners" must undergo "failure" in order to become Christian. This desert image of failure provides the framework for scripture, from Adam and Eve's exile into the penitential desert "east of Eden" to John's visionary desert isle of Patmos. It is a major theme within the Old Testament itself, where Israel's forty years in the desert are repeated as exile each time Israel becomes "successful." Moses' forty desert days preparing to receive the Law and Elijah's forty days in the desert as preparation to hear God's voice are paralleled in the New Testament by Jesus' forty wilderness days as gateway for his own ministry. And since "in every respect" he was "tempted as we are" (Heb. 4: 15), his basic temptations expose ours: power, status, and security (Matt. 4: 1-11).

With this revelation, our dilemma becomes clear. These temptations are precisely those which our society identifies as the marks of success, in the pursuit of which we have been socialized from near birth. In contrast, Jesus never once promised his disciples a suburban split-level. Instead, he called for them to leave their houses, wives, parents, children; to be mocked, shamefully treated, spit upon, scourged and killed (Luke 18: 24-34). In other words, to fail–purged of both ambition and profit.

AGING:
A SYMBOLIZATION-AVOIDANCE THEORY

Our hope, ironically, is that these three marks of "success" are what the aging process progressively threatens to take from us: our power, status and security. Such "failure" is not simply the natural result of aging but is focused by the rejective attitude of our society toward the elderly. Gerontologists recognize up to eight basic theories as to what happens to persons in modern society as they age. Yet they all miss one central factor. I call it "symbolization-avoidance."[4] The aging person, ailing and pitiful, becomes a symbol for our common fate: death. To avoid the reality of our own death, we simply corral and avoid the elderly.[5] While in Puritan days death was viewed as a glorious reunion, a birthing into eternity, it is the denial of death that marks heavily our society.[6]

In Appalachia, where I was raised, when someone showed signs of aging, we said that "Charlie is failing." To age meant to fail. Therefore, I should not have been surprised that when my father was diagnosed as having cancer, my mother hid that "failure" from everyone, including me. By the time I found out, by accident, the crisis was severe. My mother had identified herself so completely with my father's success that as he "failed," she too became a failure. Day after day she starved herself, afraid to outlast him. Although she was a faithful Christian, her intentional self-destruction witnesses that the church never taught her the kind of intentional failure that makes all things new, even when alone.

Society, too, had failed her as it does all of us. Death has become a symbol of our precarious societal condition. It reminds us that we are fallible and fragile within a society built upon "expendableness," throwaway resources built by dispensable workers. Coupled with the idea that death is proof of our ontic contingency, death takes on an uncanny power that makes it "socially unacceptable." By compartmentalization, we seek to avoid it, hospitalizing the ill, institutionalizing the aging, and pretending death away as a medical failure. In all of this, the aged person becomes imaged as the primary herald and omen of death, Cooley's "looking-glass self," eye to eye, skull to skull.

"People don't want the elderly around to remind them of their finitude. There is a centrifugal force at work, hurting older people to the circumference of life."[7] In becoming "socially non-functioning," they are quarantined so as not to be "emotionally threatening," placed in a state of "premature social extinction" so that the rest of us "can go on" with our lives.[8] That which society attempts to distance is what William May calls the "inner sense of bankruptcy." Death forces on us the fact that we are contingent nonabsolute beings and with it exposes the mortality of the myth with which our society feeds us.[9] Such avoidance has its price, however, giving to many "no alternative but to cling to life and avoid direct confrontation with the unknown."[10] Such "false consciousness" is difficult to maintain. And so it is that the "experience of one's mortality is at the core of the midlife crisis."[11]

RETIREMENT AS CONVERSATION

Because of this societal attitude, the "desert" for many of us has a gateway marked with a sign: "retirement." First a gold watch, then polite applause and life is over. Whatever we and our spouse may have done has been reduced to grist for a fading memory. The reality sinks in quickly that we are no longer needed. The word *desert* comes from *de* ("to separate") and *serere* ("to knit"). Here *desert* means "being torn from society's normal fabric." Little wonder that retirement is so traumatic, for we have been socialized to be workaholics. With self-worth defined by *doing*, having nothing to do threatens us to the core. With identity defined by job, retirement stamps us as useless, unneed-ed, and unwanted. In being "nobody," we stand on the desert's sandy edge.

Erik Erikson puts the situation well. Life's final stage begins at the juncture between despair and the struggle for integrity. The road most traveled is the one paved with despair. And we who do ministry with the aging are poor tour guides, for we betray the gospel with shuffle-board. That is, we make it our goal to keep the elderly so active that they cannot experience their failure (as defined by society). Thomas Merton pushes us to accountability, however. Spirituality, he insists, begins when a person is able to do nothing and feel no guilt. But such spirituality seems unavailable to us, for we have been programmed to the contrary: to do nothing is to feel worthless. Thus the road well traveled is not into the integrity of Christian spirituality but into the despair of "more of the same." Addicted to the process as we are, it hardly matters what we do, as long as we "stay active." "DO, DO, DO" is the chant, as we hobble up the "down" stairs.

Thus it is crucial for the church to awaken to the aging process as the desert that can bring the *spiritual conversion* which our whole society needs. It begins by facing "retirement" head-on–not calling it "redeployment" or some other euphemism. It must become what the word means, which is to pull back, take stock, and reconsider the whole with new eyes. In so doing, the despair of unrolling one's final end of string can be transformed into a new state. It is as if the best has been kept for last.

When Jesus was asked about the kingdom of God, he placed a child in their midst: "Unless you change and become like children, you will never enter the kingdom of heaven" (Matt. 18: 3). Today he might have called an older person into our midst: "Unless you go through the desert experience which society is thrusting upon these persons, you will die without having lived." The desert experience, like aging, is what our society fears and hides from like the plague. The Christian failure which transforms begins with one fact: aging is a disease for which there is no cure. Our obsession with "youth" is simply a gaudy cover for our best-kept secret that each of us will fail, totally, and that the unraveling will stretch well over half a lifetime.

The real question for Christians is not whether we will fail, but whether we will live our failure intentionally, choosing it before the end. Crucial, then, is the conversion of motivation, for the gauge of Christian spirituality is giving without expectation of return, turning gladly one's other cheek when struck, and embracing our enemy as friend. The story is told of the desert father who ran after the robbers who had pillaged his cell to give them something they had overlooked. The desert experience illustrated here teaches us that we cannot be Christian by our own efforts. Such spirituality dare not be the "sour grapes" of not wanting power, status, and security because one is not able to get them. Instead there must be that redemptive process through which the very craving for culture's "values" is broken. Life blossoms when "we find ourselves willing to be last, not because the last may become first, but because the game of 'firsts' and 'lasts' is no longer of interest."[12]

"Where," asked T.S. Eliot, "is the Life we have lost in living?" True, Life is not at center a matter of *doing* at all, but of *being*. Here the God-intended affinity between children and the elderly is touched in the simple and thankful joy of being alive. But how can one relearn to savor each moment for its own intrinsic sake? It begins with retirement's "ontic shock" that society can get along much better without me.[13] Then the other side is born: the discovery that I can get along much better without those societal values on the basis of which I have been rendered dispensable.

As ministers to the aging, we have the incredible responsibility as spiritual directors to do what the church should have been doing all along. After sixty plus years of drivenness, what needs to happen is nothing short of conversion. For perhaps the first time, one must be opened to glory in *being* simply in being *alive* without need to do or act or succeed or justify in any way one's life. *The name for such living is grace.*

Aging evokes this desert spirituality when sometime, somewhere, everything is "up for grabs."[14] This point of no return is most likely to occur when one's life string feels very short. "Is this all there is?" With this question, the desire for power, status, and security whose craving has pushed us for a lifetime takes on a hollow ache. With the end in sight, "more and more" takes on the feeling of "less and less." Why? Way down deep we know what we have spent a lifetime hiding, because we have not, nor can we ever, justify our being by our doing. Whatever sense of competence or achievement we might have gained as down payment on acceptability, the aging process turns to mush, day by day, until retirement or death, whichever comes first. Naked we come into the world, and naked we will leave, no matter how many possessions are piled around us on our bed. Real meaning resides neither in doing nor having, but in the integrity of life drunk deeply, intrinsically, thankfully.

SIN AS TAKING FOR GRANTED

At its core, sin is the arrogance of taking things for granted. To see one moon is to see them all. Each day is like every day, *ad infinitum, ad absurdum.* "All things are weariness . . . [for] what has been done is what will be done; and there is nothing new under the sun" (Eccles. 1: 8-9). The desert conversion begins when, in running out of time, one is brought face to face with the foundational truth about every moment of life. Each second I am one heartbeat away from oblivion one breath away, one anything away, from death. And in living fully that truth, one's life can be transformed by living each moment *as if it were the final one.* Resurrection becomes the ongoing gift of one new day at a time.

This can be illustrated. Picture yourself on death row. After years of appeals, the judge has ruled: today you will die. Everything from this point on will be the last time. The last bite of roast beef, the final sip of coffee ever. Sixteen paces to the electric chair. Step by step. Until the final one ever. The cold leather straps. Swallowing for a last time. The final look of color, the green shade. Counting breaths five, four, three.

The telephone rings. The Governor. Let him go! Reprieve! Free, my God; I'm free at last! Through the huge metal doors out into the sunlight, down the front steps, three at a time. Never has blue sky been bluer! Wet green grass against warm bare feet. Smiles and waves, to everyone, up and down the street. Eyes. Beautiful. Straight to McDonald's for the largest orange juice ever poured. And there to drink as libation to the whole of creation. AH-THE BLOOD OF CHRIST![15]

We have reached the mysterious heart of desert spirituality. *To live every moment as if it were the last is to savor each part of life as though it were the first*. Here it is. The last and the first merge, the beginning restored as the end and "the end is where we start from." Pablo Picasso was right: It takes a long, long time to become young. One becomes flooded with the taste of "first times": when first one fell in love, or made a July snowball in the Rocky Mountains, or tasted with surprise the salty surf. James Fowler identifies this stage, occurring after the "sacrament of defeat," as a "second naiveté."[16] Sam Keen calls it the lifestyle of the "foolish lover."[17] All depends on the paradox of contingency where in facing the finality of aging one receives back each speck of life as gift. One day at a time, one hour at a time, thankful for quaffing each moment for its own dear sake. Resurrection has meaning, Barth insisted, only for those so in love with creation that they grieve at the thought of leaving. Ironic though it sounds *aging* can bring this ecstasy over the commonplace a whippoorwill in spring, wind through fall willows, vibrant color adorning one's bedspread, the twitch of energy to an arthritic finger. On the night before his execution, Camus's hero heard the evening sounds coming through a crack in his prison wall. Almost too late he learned. It is possible to live in one moment more than most persons live in a lifetime.[18]

Jesus rooted this mystery of desert spirituality in the forfeiting of anxiety, in taking no thought of the morrow but living each new day as sufficient unto itself (Luke 12: 22ff.). Most of us squander our days, permitting the future to play havoc with each present. In kindergarten, I could not wait to be old enough for knickers, then long pants, to get a license to drive; life would begin when I graduated; or is it with my first job? Perhaps when I get married, or will it be with the first child, or when the last one finally leaves home? Certainly when I retire, or at least by the time . . . I die? "I do not want to get to the end," said Thoreau, "and find that I have never lived." Yet nothing seems able to stop us from living life as means rather than as end except being shaken profoundly by the nearness of an end whereby there will be no later."[19]

There is a sundial in front of my hermitage. On it the words are old, the writing worn, the meaning clear.

> *Grow old along with me.*
> *The best is yet to be.*

REFERENCES

1. Stanley Hauerwas, *The Peaceable Kingdom* (South Bend: University of Notre Dame Press, 1983), 27.

2. Ibid., 68.

3. W. Paul Jones, "Intentional Failure: The Importance of the Desert Experience," *Weavings*, vol. VII, no. 1, January/February 1992, 16-22.

4. W. Paul Jones, "Death as a Factor in Understanding Modern Attitudes Toward the Aging: A Symbolization-Avoidance Theory," David B. Oliver ed., *New Directions in Religion and Aging* (New York: The Haworth Press, Inc. 1987), 75-90.

5. David Stannard, *The Puritan Way of Death* (New York: Oxford, 1977).

6. Ernest Becker, *The Denial of Death* (New York: The Free Press, 1973).

7. Eugene Bianchi, "Aging as a Spiritual Journey," JSAC *Grapevine, 15* (Nov. 1983), 2.

8. Stannard, *The Puritan Way*, 194.

9. Bianchi, "Aging as a Spiritual Journey," 2.

10. Stannard, *The Puritan Way, 194.*

11. Daniel J. Levinson, et al., *The Seasons of a Man's Life (New York: Alfred A. Knopf, 1978), 26.*

12. Jones, "Intentional Failure," 22.

13. Cf. Paul Tillich, *Systematic Theology* (Chicago: University of Chicago, 1951), I:113.

14. See Charles Cummings, "Job's Desert Experience," *Studies in Formative Spirituality*, vol. I, no. 2, 227-236. Also Charles Cummings, *Spirituality and Desert Experience* (Ann Arbor: University Microfilms International, 1977).

15. For the scope of such a spirituality rooted in the aging process, see W. Paul Jones, "Aging as a Spiritualizing Process," *Journal of Religion and Aging*, vol. 1, no. 1 (Fall 1984): 3-16. Also W. Paul Jones, "Theology and Aging in the 21st Century," in Oliver, *New Directions in Religion and Aging, 17-32.*

16. James Fowler, *Stages of Faith* (San Francisco: Harper and Row, 1981), 198.

17. James Fowler and Sam Keen, *Life Maps: Conversations on the Journey of Faith* (Waco: Word Books, 1978).

18. Albert Camus, *The Stranger* (New York: Alfred A. Knoph, 1946), 136.

19. For a development of the values contrasting the perspective of "doing" and "being," see W. Paul Jones, "Gerontology: Spirituality and Aging," in *Quarterly Papers on Religion and Aging*, Oubri A. Poppele Center for Health and Welfare Ministries, vol. 1, no. 1, (Summer 1984), 2-3.

Index

© 2001 by The Haworth Press, Inc. All rights reserved.